DRUGS

G L David Krupadanam • D Vijaya Prasad
K Varaprasad Rao • K L N Reddy
C Sudhakar

Universities Press

DRUGS

UNIVERSITIES PRESS (INDIA) PRIVATE LIMITED

Registered Office
3-6-747/1/A & 3-6-754/1, Himayatnagar, Hyderabad 500 029, Telangana, India
info@universitiespress.com, www.universitiespress.com

Distributed by
Orient Blackswan Private Limited

Registered Office
3-6-752, Himayatnagar, Hyderabad 500 029, Telangana, India

Other Offices
Bengaluru, Chennai, Guwahati, Hyderabad,
Kolkata, Mumbai, New Delhi, Noida, Patna

First published 2001
Reprinted 2004, 2016, 2022, 2023

ISBN 978-81-7371-386-6

Typeset in Life BT 10/12 *by*
Orient BlackSwan, Hyderabad 500 039

Printed in India by
Replika Press Pvt. Ltd., Kundli Sonepat 131 028, Haryana

Published by
Universities Press (India) Private Limited
3-6-747/1/A & 3-6-754/1, Himayatnagar, Hyderabad 500 029, Telangana, India

Contents

Preface

Drugs have played a central role in the progress of human civilization. Primitive man depended mainly on plant products and metal salts to cure diseases, while modern man uses a wide range of synthetic organic compounds and biotechnology-derived vaccines, antibiotics, etc.

There are many important stages before a compound is used as a drug to treat a disease. The first stage is drug discovery, where several thousands of compounds are screened and evaluated for their efficacy and the best is selected. The second stage is the manufacture of the drug using well-understood chemistry and adapting safe and clean manufacturing, analytical practices. The third stage is the formulation of the drug in a convenient dosage form as tablets, capsules, injections and solutions. There are some drugs that have been discovered serendipitously as in the case of the antibiotic, penicillin. Some plant-derived drugs have been known to man from very early times, like quinine, ephedrine, cocaine, and morphine, which are extensively used even today.

This book deals with the historical aspects of the development and use of drugs, vitamins, hormones and their classification, formulations and the general principles of drug action. The pharmacokinetics, the interaction of drugs at the targeted receptor with special reference to the agonist, antagonist, enzyme inhibitior and antimetabolites, are discussed. The drugs acting on the central and autonomic nervous systems, cardiac agents, hematopoietic agents and diuretics are dealt with at length. The structure–activity relationships are described and the chemistry involved in synthesis of drugs is also explained in detail.

This book is meant for B.Sc. chemistry students in all Indian universities, as well as those working in R & D laboratories of drug and pharmaceutical industries. Chemists play a key role in pharmaceutical research, as they synthesize, purify and analyze drugs. This book is designed to help chemists with little or no knowledge of commonly used drugs.

In order to make the contents as clear as possible, even to a beginner, the subject matter has been presented in a comprehensive, systematic and lucid manner, using simple language. Special care has been taken in the preparation of the drawings, tables and schemes. Long and short answer questions, a bibliography and a glossary have been provided for the benefit of students. We are aware that there is scope for improvement in this book and welcome critical suggestions.

Several of our colleagues have inspired us to take up the task of writing this book and assisted us in more ways than one in the preparation of this book and we are beholden to all of them. We are particularly grateful to Dr. S. Janaki Rani, Reader in Botany, Government City College, Hyderabad and Dr. Durga Prasad Sunkara, M.D., Houston, USA, with whom we have had long discussions which have helped us immensely. We also thank Dr. B. Parthasaradhi Reddy, Chairman, Hetero Drugs Ltd., Hyderabad, for his cooperation and assistance in bringing out this book. We owe a special debt of gratitude to our friends Mr. Madhu Reddy and Ms. Chandini Rao for going through the manuscript and improving the drafts.

Our sincere thanks are due to Universities Press (I) Ltd. and Messrs. Orient Longman for evincing keen interest in publishing this book. We are thankful to Mr. M. Nayab for his assiduous services in typesetting and drawing, and Mr. C. Debdaan for the cover design.

G.L. David Krupadanam

D. Vijaya Prasad

K. Varaprasad Rao

K.L.N. Reddy

C. Sudhakar

1 INTRODUCTION

Drugs cure disease. Drugs, in the form of plant products and minerals, have been used from times immemorial. Initially, nature itself provided the therapeutic agents. Primitive man discovered appropriate cures for various ailments through trial and error by chewing plant products such as roots, bark, leaves and fruits, and this information was passed on to subsequent generations by word of mouth. Today, drugs are employed to reduce pain, fever, acidity, blood pressure, mental depression, etc., or to combat infectious diseases. Drugs may be used to diagnose diabetes, liver malfunction, pregnancy; or they may be employed to replenish a deficiency in antibodies, vitamins, hormones, electrolytes or proteins and enzymes. They may also be used to prevent pregnancy, or to assist the maintenance of pregnancy, or to extend life itself. Drugs can leave residual effects after administration has ceased. Drugs can conceal disease as well. Broadly, a **disease can be defined as an endogenous biochemical imbalance, an abnormal and aberrant proliferation of cells, or an exogenous chemical toxin or an invasive pathogen in the body**.

The word **drug** is derived from French word 'drogue' which means a 'dry herb'. **A drug is defined as an agent intended for use in the diagnosis, mitigation, treatment, cure or prevention of disease in man or in other animals.** One of the most astounding qualities of drugs is the diversity of their actions and effects on the body. According to World Health Organisation (WHO), who promote basic health globally, **"A drug is any substance or product that is used or intended to be used to modify or explore physiological systems or pathological states for the benefit of the recipient."**

How drugs act and interact, how they enter the body tissue, what happens to them inside the body, how they are eliminated from it, and the effects of genetics, age and disease on drug action, are all important to the scientists who discover the drugs and also to the people who use the drugs. There are risks in not taking medicines when they are needed and there are also risks in using medicines indiscriminately. Drugs have to be applied correctly, in a proper dosage, for a specific period of time in relation not only to properties of the drugs, but also to those of the patient and the disease. William Withering, who defined the use of *Digitalis* (foxglove leaves) in heart disorders, wrote in 1787,

> ...poisons in small doses are the best medicines and useful medicines in too large doses are poisonous, i.e., drugs are useful poisons.

The vast array of effective drugs available today represent one of man's greatest scientific accomplishments. It would be frightening to conceive of our civilization devoid of these remarkable and beneficial drugs. Through their use, many of the diseases which have plagued mankind throughout history, such as smallpox and poliomyelitis, are now virtually extinct. Chronic illnesses, such as diabetes, hypertension and mental depression, are now effectively controlled with modern drugs. Today's surgical procedures would be virtually impossible without the benefit of general anaesthetics, analgesics, antibiotics, blood transfusions and intravenous fluids and nutrients.

The process of discovery of a drug and its development is complex. It involves the collective contributions of many scientific specialists, such as organic, physical and analytical chemists, biochemists, bacteriologists, physiologists, pharmacologists, toxicologists, hematologists, immunologists, endocrinologists, pathologists, pharmaceutical scientists, clinical physicians, and many others.

1.1 The requirements of an ideal drug

Until the 19th century, diseases were cured simply by using extracts of roots, barks, herbs and animal parts. Different drug substances, because of their unique chemical structures, exert their own individual effects on the biological system. In general, drugs exert their effects:

(a) by modifying the biochemical or metabolic process of the body's cells or enzyme functions. For example, aspirin (1), omeprazole (2), captopril, ibuprofen, etc.

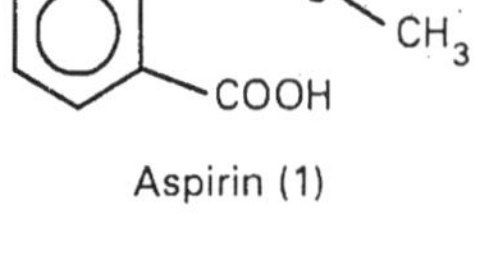

Aspirin (1)

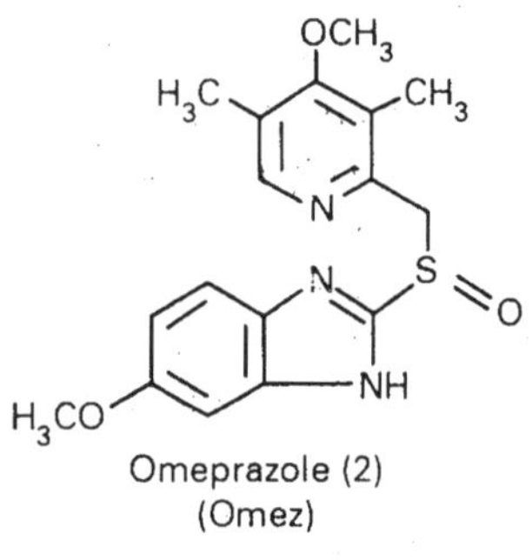

Omeprazole (2)
(Omez)

(b) by modifying the metabolic activity of invading pathogens, as antibiotics. For example, penicillin, streptomycin, gentamycin, etc.
(c) by reacting chemically, as antacids that reduce excess gastric acidity. For example, gelusil, digene, etc.
(d) by physical action, as the protective effects of ointments upon topical application. For example, burnol, silverex, etc.

An ideal drug should possess the following requirements:

1. It should produce the specifically desired effect.
2. The action of the drug should be localized at the site where it is desired to act (site specificity).
3. Be administered by the most desired route (generally orally) at minimal dosage and dosing frequency.
4. It should exhibit no side effects.
5. It should eliminate the disease from the body efficiently, completely, and without residual effect.
6. It should be non-toxic.
7. The drug should not injure or damage the host tissues or physiological processes.
8. It should not make the host cells resistant to the drug after its use, for some time. (In actual practice, the cells which were originally susceptible to the action of a particular drug may, after some time, acquire a tolerance or resistance to that drug.)
9. It should be available everywhere.
10. It should be easily produced, at low cost.
11. It should be pharmaceutically elegant, and physically and chemically stable under various conditions of use and storage.
12. It should be manufactured by or with the approval of the Government, as per the specifications.

However, these qualities and features are still far away from realization for a majority of the commonly used drugs.

1.2 Sources of drugs

Drugs are discovered from a variety of natural sources or created synthetically in the laboratory, as a result of many years of tireless research. There are, however, a few cases where the drugs were discovered accidentally. The sources of drugs include: (1) plant origin drugs, (2) animal origin drugs, (3) synthetic drugs, (4) biotechnology and (5) human gene therapy.

1.2.1 Plant origin drugs

Throughout history, plant materials have served as a reservoir of potential new drugs. Only a very small portion of the plant species so far identified, have been investigated for medicinal agents. Certain major contributions to modern drug therapy may be attributed to the successful conversion of botanic folklore remedies into modern wonder drugs. Reserpine (3), a tranquillizer and hypotensive agent, is an example of a medicine isolated from the folklore remedy of the plant *Rauwolfia serpentina*. Another plant drug, Periwinkle or *Vinca Rosea*, was scientifically investigated as a result of its reputation in folklore as an useful agent in the treatment of diabetes melitus. But now, two alkaloids, vincristine and vinblastine, have been isolated from this plant and are used as anti-cancer drugs. After the isolation and structural identification of active plant constituents, organic chemists may recreate them by total synthesis in the laboratory or, more importantly, use the natural chemical as the starting material in the creation of slightly different chemical structures by means of molecule manipulation.The new structures, termed 'semisynthetic drugs,' may have a slightly or vastly different pharmacological activity from that of the starting substance, depending upon the nature and extent of chemical alteration. Plant constituents which may be inactive or rather unimportant therapeutically, may be employed in the semi-synthetic process to yield important drugs, with profound pharmacological activity. For example, the various species of *Dioscorea* are rich in steroids from which hormonal drugs like cortisone and estrogens, the female sex hormones, are semisynthetically produced.

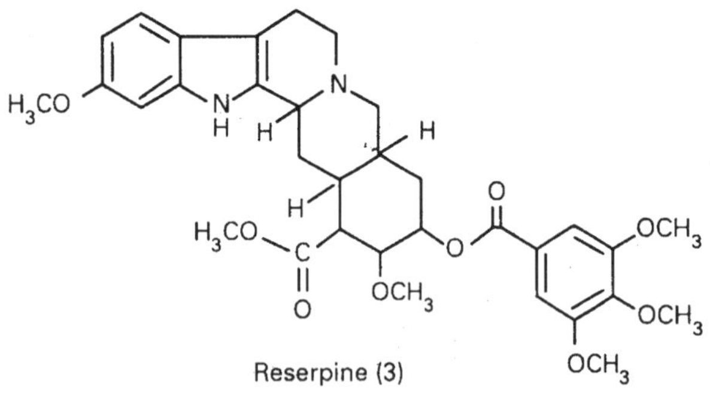

Reserpine (3)

1.2.2 Animal origin drugs

Animals have served humans in their search for drugs in a number of ways. They not only have yielded to drug testing and biologic assay procedures, but also have provided drugs from their own tissues or through their biological processes. Hormonal substances such as thyroid extract, insulin and the pituitary hormone, obtained from the endocrine glands of cattle, sheep and swine, are life-saving drugs employed daily as replacement therapy in the human body. The urine of pregnant mares is a rich source of estrogens. The use of animals in the production of various biological products, including serums, antitoxins and vaccines, has been of life-saving significance ever since the pioneering work of Dr Edward Jenner on the smallpox vaccine in England in 1796. Today, the poliomyelitis vaccine is prepared in cultures of rhesus monkey tissue, the mumps and influenza vaccines in fluids of chick embryos, the rubella (German measles) vaccine in duck embryos and the smallpox vaccine from the skin of bovine calves. Tomorrow, vaccines for diseases like AIDS and cancer may be developed through the utilization of cell and tissue cultures.

1.2.3 Synthetic drugs

Today, the most common source of potential drugs is the laboratory. Scientists, through their skill, are creating not only chemical modifications of known structures but also totally new synthetic organic compounds. Spectacular successes have been achieved in the field of synthetic drugs in the last 100 years. The structure of the synthesized drug, generally, is similar to that of the natural drug. In fact, the synthesized drug should have a simpler structure than that of a natural drug. The aim is that a synthesized drug should have more useful properties than the natural drug. For instance, Novocain (4), a synthetic anesthetic, has a simpler structure with no side effects compared to cocaine (5) which has a more complex structure and many side effects.

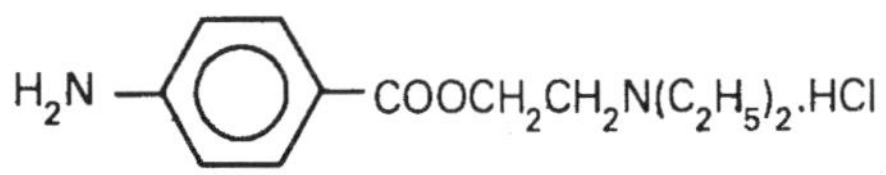

Novocain (4)
(Procaine hydrochloride)

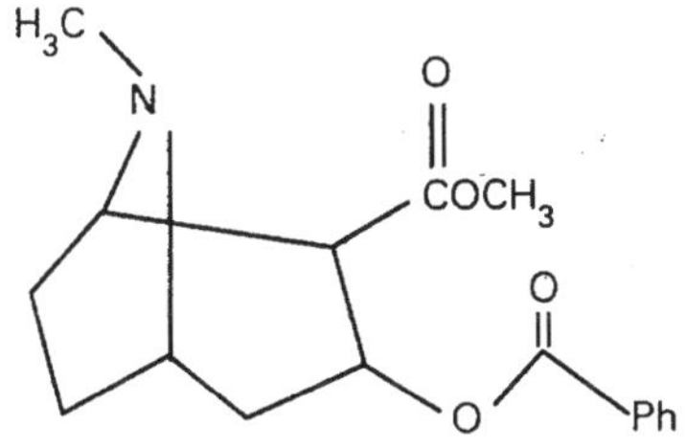

Cocaine (5)

A majority of drugs used today are of synthetic origin. Anesthetic drugs like thiopental sodium (6), and methohexital, sedative drugs like benzodiazepines and phenobarbital (7), antipyretic drugs like aspirin (1) and phenylbutazone (8), analgesic drugs like paracetamol (9) and analgin (10), anti-inflammatory drugs like ibuprofen (11), anticonvulsants like diazepam (12) and gabapentin, bronchodilators like salbutamol,

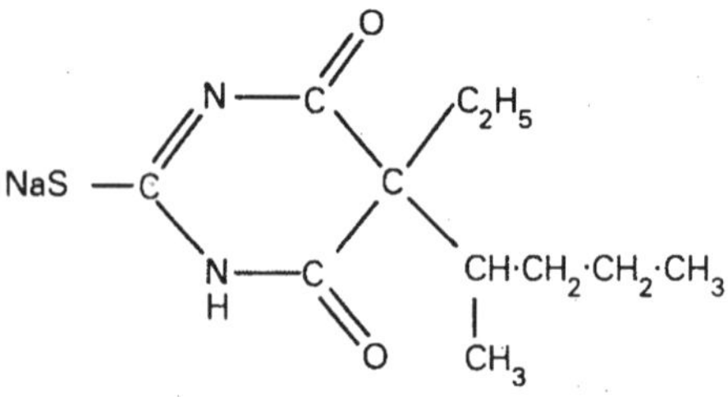

Thiopental sodium (6)

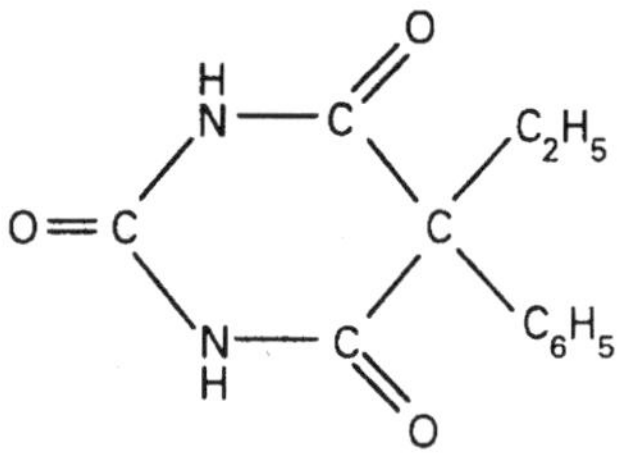

Phenobarbital (7)
(Luminal)

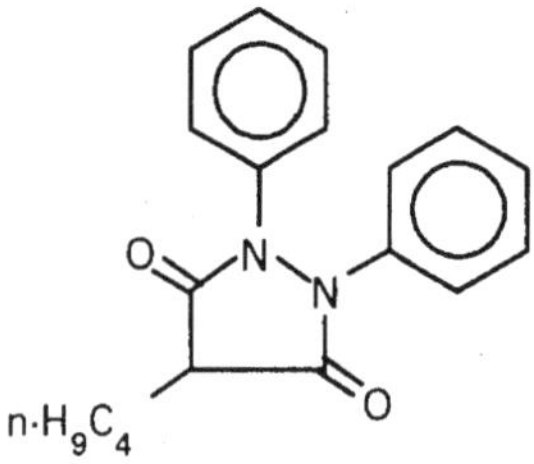

Phenylbutazone (8)
(Butazolidin)

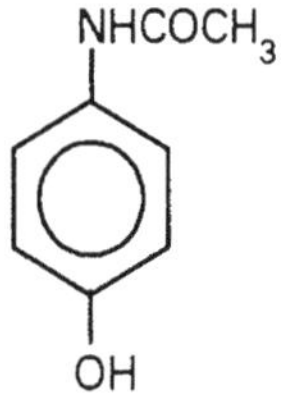

Paracetamol (9)

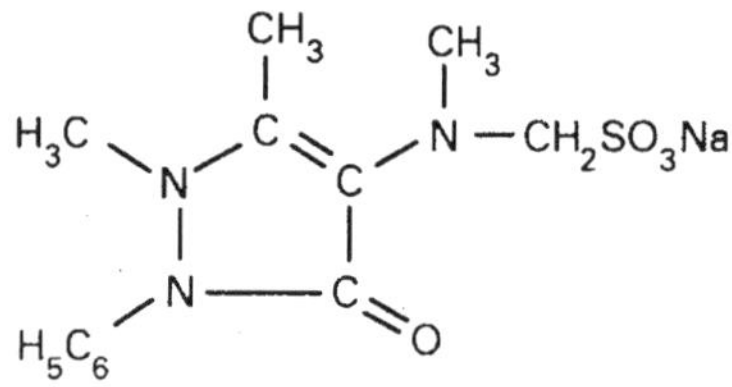

Analgin (10)
(Novalgin)

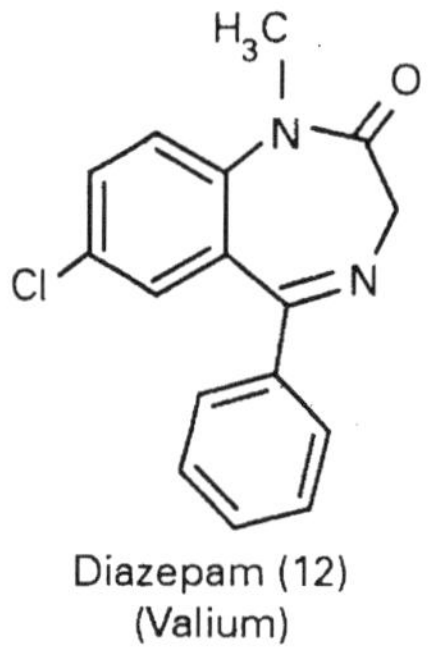

Diazepam (12)
(Valium)

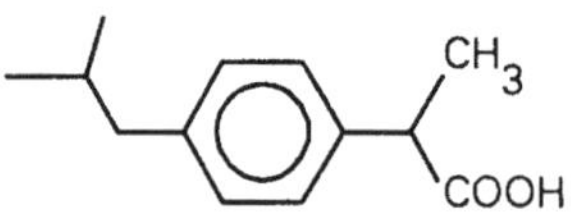

Ibuprofen (11)

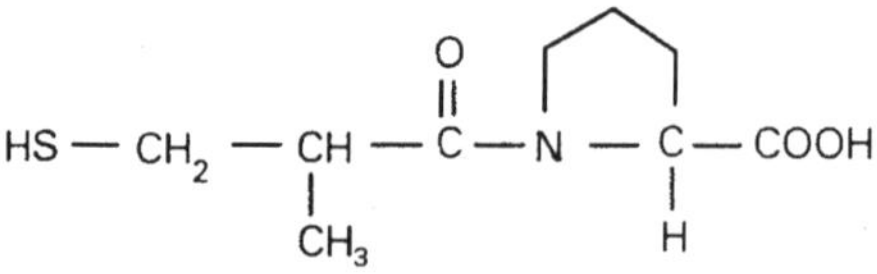

Captopril (13)

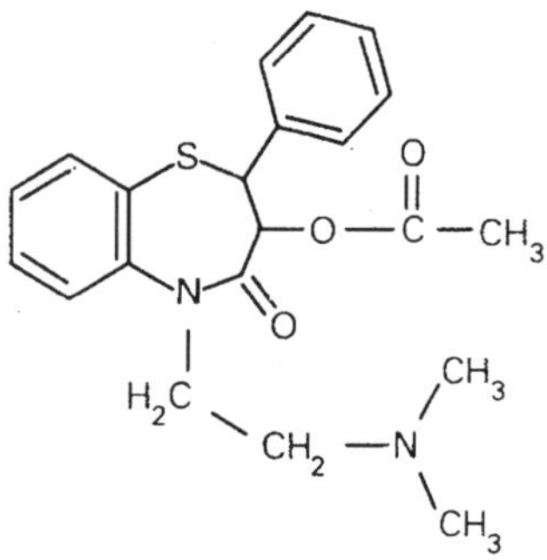

Diltiazem (14)

antihypertensive drugs like captopril (13) and guanethidine, and cardiovascular drugs like diltiazem (14), and cardene, are just a few examples from the vast array of synthetic compounds.

1.2.4 Biotechnology

Today, we are witnessing a new era in the development of pharmaceutical products due to the advent of genetic engineering, the submicroscopic manipulation of the "double helix," the spiral DNA chain of life. Through this process, more abundant and much purer antibiotics, vaccines and biological products can be produced to combat human diseases. There are two basic technologies in the genetic field of drug development. They are recombinant DNA (r DNA) and monoclonal antibody (Mo AB) production. What is common to both techniques is the ability to manipulate and produce proteins, the building blocks of living matter. Proteins represent an almost infinite source of drugs. They are made up of long chains of amino acids, and their sequence and spatial configuration offer a staggering number of possibilities. Both recombinant DNA and monoclonal antibody production techniques influence cells in their ability to produce proteins. The more fundamental of the two techniques is the recombinant DNA. It can potentially produce almost any protein. It is possible to transplant genetic material from higher species such as man into lower species like bacterium. This so-called "gene splicing" can induce the lower organism to make proteins it would not have made otherwise. Drugs such as human insulin, human growth hormone, hepatitis B vaccine, epoetin alpha, and interferon are being produced in this manner.

While the recombinant DNA technique involves the manipulation of proteins within the cells of lower animals, the monoclonal antibody production is conducted entirely within the cells of higher animals, including the patient. The technique exploits the ability of the cells to produce a desired antibody, and stimulates pure antibody production. These antibodies then have the capacity to combat the specific target. Monoclonal antibodies have enormous potential to change the face of medicine and pharmacy in the next decade, and applications for their use are already in progress. In medicine, monoclonal antibodies are being used to localize malignant cancer cells, and it is anticipated that they will be used in the future to combat diseases like juvenile onset of diabetes.

1.2.5 Human gene therapy

Human gene therapy, used to prevent, treat, cure, diagnose, or mitigate human diseases caused by genetic disorders, represents another promising new technology. Gene therapy is a medical intervention based on the modification of the genetic material of living cells. Cells may be modified outside the body (*in vitro*) for subsequent administration, or they may be modified within the body (*in vivo*) by gene therapy products given directly to the patient. In both cases, gene therapy involves the transfer of new genetic material to the cells of a patient afflicted with a genetic disease. The genetic material, usually cloned DNA, may be transferred into the patient's cells physically through micro-injection, or chemically mediated transfer procedures that integrate genetic material directly into the host cell chromosomes. Gene therapy is being examined for a number of genetic-based blood and immunological diseases like sickle cell anemia, Cooley's anemia, malignant melanoma and renal cell cancer. Recent advances seem to offer promise for the future.

1.3 *Historical evolution of drugs*

The use of drugs undoubtedly dates beyond recorded history. The instinct of primitive man to relieve the pain of a wound by bathing it in cool water or soothing it with a fresh leaf or protecting it with the application of mud or animal excreta, is all within the scope of superstition and belief. Ancient man ascribed disease to divine wrath and other supernatural powers. Among many early races, disease was believed to be caused by the entry of demons or evil spirits into the body. The wise man or woman of the tribe, whose knowledge of the healing qualities of plants had been gathered through experience or handed down from generation to generation by word of mouth, was called upon to attend to the sick or wounded. It was in the preparation of the medicinal materials that the art of the 'apothecary' (old name for one who prepares and sells drugs, now chemist) originated. The practitioners were believed to have a connection with the world of spirits and, thus, played the role of intermediaries between the seen and the unseen. The belief that drugs had magical associations, made their natural qualities irrelevant. The compassion of God, the observance of ceremonies, the absence of evil spirits and the healing intent of the dispenser were individually and collectively necessary to make the drug effective. From historical records, it is evident that the knowledge of drugs and their application to disease has always implied the possession of some supernatural power.

In the Homeric epics, the Greek term *pharmakon*, from which the word *pharmacy* was derived, connotes a drug that can be used for good or for evil purposes. As time passed, the art of the apothecary became combined with priestly functions. Among the early civilizations, the 'priest-physician' became the healer of the body as well as of the soul. The use of *digitalis*, an

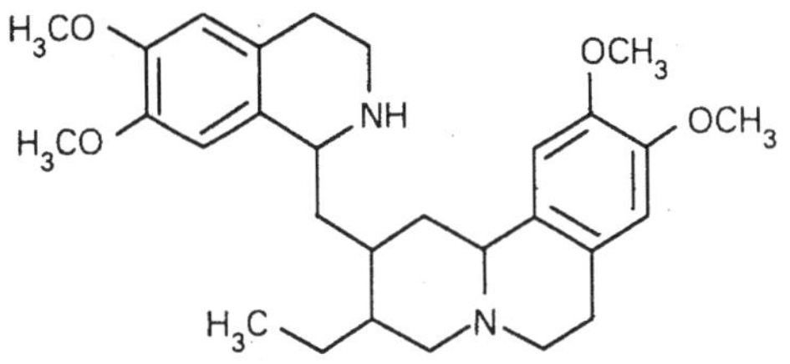

Emetine (15)

extract of foxglove leaves, for the treatment of dropsy (i.e., heart disorders) was known to the early man. The *ipecacuahna* root which was used for the treatment of dysentery and diarrhoea contains the alkaloid, emetine (15), which is an important drug in the treatment of amoebiasis even today.

The world's oldest known pharmacological or therapeutic writings came from India and China. The earliest Indian records are the *Vedas*. The medicinal properties of plants are described in the *Rigveda* and *Atharvaveda* (3500–1500 BC), from which Ayurveda (knowledge of life or the science of life) was developed. Throughout history many individuals have contributed to the advancement of the health sciences, whose genius and creativeness had a revolutionary influence on the development of pharmacy and medicine. It was Charaka, a renowned ancient Indian physician, and later Sushruta and Vagbhatta, who described various medicinal preparations in Ayurveda. The ***Charakasamhita*** dealing mostly with plants and ***Sushrutsamhita*** dealing with surgery, are the best-known ancient treatises in Ayurveda. The efficacy of *Amla* fruit as a tonic, the use of *Rauwolfia serpentina* as a tranquillizer and to treat insanity, the anti-leprotic action of the *Chaulmoogra* fruit, the dried roots and stems of *Withania somnifera* (Aswangandha) as a sedative were known to ancient Indians. Charaka described about 300 vegetable drugs and classified them according to their effects, mostly symptoms, into 50 groups.

The antipyretic effects of Ch'ang Shang, which has now been shown to contain antimalarial alkaloids, and the drug 'Ma Huang' for its diaphoretic and stimulatory effect, were discovered by Chinese Emperor-Scholar Shen Nung (2735 BC). The great herbal or Chinese materia medica, ***Pan Tsao*** was probably written in 2735 BC and contains many vegetable and metallic preparations and a few animal products including toad's eyelids, elephant's and tiger's bones, and other such material as horns and fins. The oldest records of medicinal plants were also found in the Mediterranean civilizations of the Greeks, Romans, Hebrews and Egyptians. The *Papyri* were the first written accounts of medicinal experiences from Egypt. The Papyrus (scroll), discovered by Eber in 1872, was prepared in 1500 BC and mentions about 700 herbal remedies, including opium. A Babylonian clay tablet (700 BC) has also been discovered, which mentions 300 different drugs.

Modern medicine is considered to date from Hippocrates, a Greek physician (450 BC) who, for the first time, rationalized medicine, systematized medical knowledge and elevated the practice of medicine to a high, ethical plane. Dioscorides (1st century AD), another Greek physician and botanist, was the first to deal with botany as the applied science of pharmacy. His work, ***De Materia Medica,*** is considered a milestone in the development of pharmaceutical botany and in the study of naturally-occuring medicinal material. Cladius Galen, a Greek pharmacist-physician who attained Roman citizenship, formulated several medicines that were followed for 1500 years. He originated so many preparations of vegetable drugs that the area of pharmaceutical preparations was once commonly referred to as 'Galenic pharmacy.' Paracelsus (1493–1541 AD), a Swiss physician and chemist, extolled the virtues of antimony salts as medicines and, for a period, metal therapy dominated over herbal rercipes.

The synthesis of phenacetin as an analgesic (pain killer) in 1889, and aspirin (1) in 1899 as an antipyretic (to reduce fever) are, perhaps, the earliest efforts to find a new source of drugs based on synthetic organic chemistry. Early research, to find synthetic drugs, was focussed on anaesthetics (ether, chloroform), hypnotics (chloral hydrate, paraldehyde), and analgesics (phenacetin, aspirin).

The pioneering work of Paul Ehrlich, the German bacteriologist and organic chemist (1854–1915), led to the emergence of chemotherapeutic drugs. The greatest impact in medicine was made by Louis Pasteur's

Gerhard Domagk, a German scientist, was testing certain drugs, for their effect on germs in rats, in the early 1930s. His daughter accidentally cut her finger with a needle while playing and infection set in. Every attempt was made, including surgery, to stop the spread of the deadly infection, but all failed. The doctors declared that there was no hope. In desperation, Domagk gave his little girl oral doses of one of the dyes that he was testing. Her fever dropped quickly and she recovered soon. Domagk had previously discovered that the dye, a sulfa compound patented under the name of Prontosil, would cure infected mice and rabbits with no harmful side-effects to the animals. Domagk's work attracted many researchers and, within a few years, a number of sulfa drugs were prepared and tested. As a tribute to his pioneering work in the synthesis of sulfa drugs, Domagk was selected for the 1939 Nobel Prize in Medicine, but Hitler prohibited Domagk from accepting it.

(1822–95) development of a vaccine for hydrophobia (rabies). The medical field has been revolutionized by the phenomenal success of sulfa drugs and antibiotics. Sulfa drugs such as prontosil (16), sulphanilamide (17), and sulphadiazine (18), were the first compounds in the early 1930s, found effective against bacterial diseases such as tuberculosis, pneumonia and diphtheria.

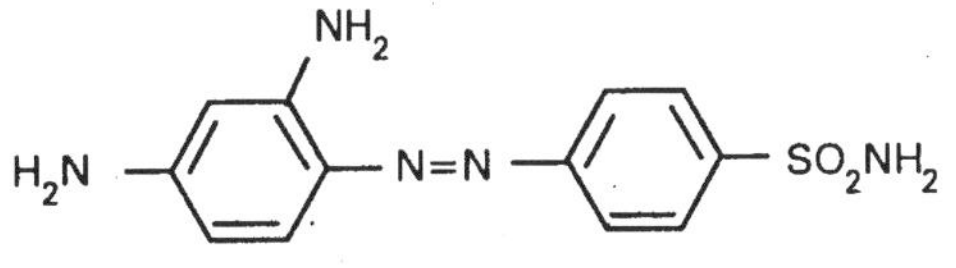

Prontosil (16)

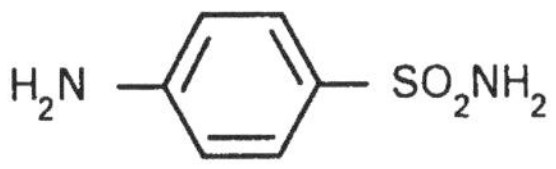

Sulphanilamide (17)

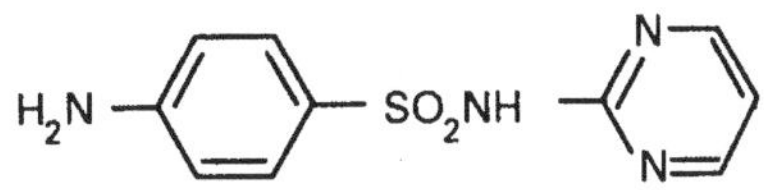

Sulphadiazine (18)

The discovery of antibiotics, the wonder drugs, was a boon to mankind. Bacteria, the simplest of free-living organisms, produce some of the most lethal poisons known to man. For example, Botulinum toxin produces respiratory paralysis, Tetanus toxin produces muscular spasm, Diphtheria toxin damages the heart, and the toxins of Staphylococci rupture red blood corpuscles. Bacteria and fungi also often produce substances that are toxic to other microorganisms but not to man and these substances, known as antibiotics, have been a therapeutic gold-mine. Penicillin was the first antibiotic to be discovered by Alexander Fleming in 1929 AD. The first successful clinical trial of crude penicillin in 1941, and the requirements of wartime, led to the discovery of a number of antibiotics such as streptomycin (1943), chloramphenicol (1947), chlorotetracycline (1948), neomycin (1949), erythromycin (1952), ampicillin (19), amoxicillin (20) and many more, earning that period a lasting place in history as the "antibiotic age".

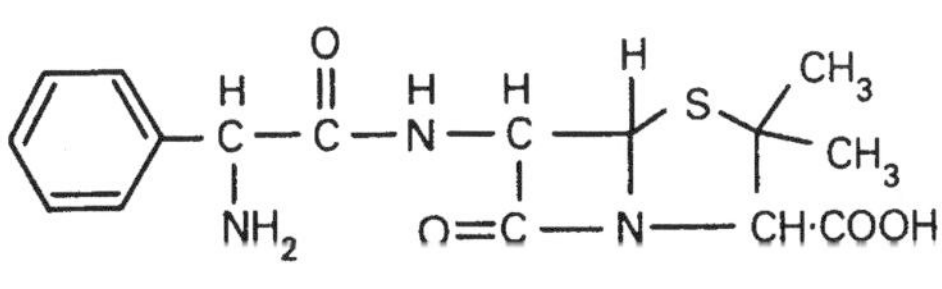

Ampicillin (19)

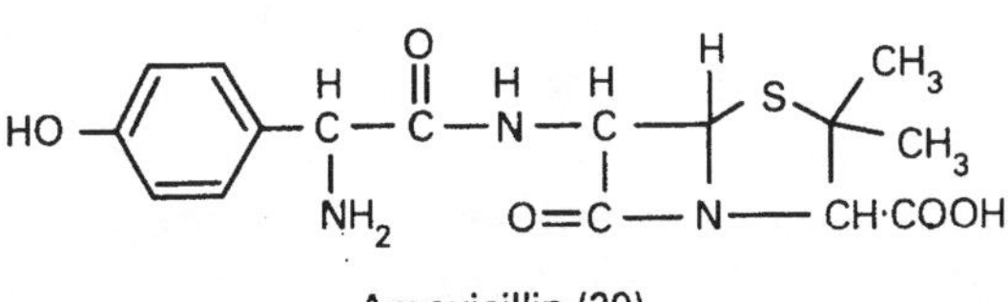

Amoxicillin (20)

It is interesting to know about the discovery of antibiotics. A British bacteriologist, Alexander Fleming, had been cultivating various bacteria in dishes. One morning, in 1929, Fleming observed that the bacteria in one dish were normal except for a spot of blue-green mould (fungi). At that spot (area) all the bacteria had died. Fleming cultivated the mould and extracted a solution, which he referred to as penicillin. He found that penicillin was very effective against pneumonia germs in mice. His findings, when published, received little attention for about 10 years. Inspired by Fleming's work, two scientists, Florey and Chain, worked at Oxford University to obtain penicillin and to try it on human beings. On February 12, 1941, the first dose of penicillin was given to a human patient. A policeman in London cut his chin while shaving and got a blood infection. He developed a burning fever and his face was swollen. Sulfa drugs were tried with no success. At this stage, for the first time, an injection of penicillin was given to the dying policeman. His temperature dropped to normal, and he was on the road to recovery. At that stage, unfortunately, the supply of penicillin was exhausted. The infection flared up again and the patient died. After some months, fresh penicillin was tried on a boy with infection that did not respond to any other treatment. The boy recovered and the power of penicillin was proved. After that, the mass production of antibiotics was taken up. The period, from 1930–1945, witnessed the most significant advancement in medicine and public health in history with the rise of sulfa drugs and antibiotics.

The early 1980s witnessed the products of modern pharmaceutical biotechnology. The recombinant DNA-produced insulin was first marketed in 1982 and, since then, the biotechnology drug-wave has been riding high. It appears almost certain that the 21st century will be dominated by the medicines generated through biotechnology and genetic engineering.

1.4 Terminology and description of the terms

1.4.1 Pharmacology

Pharmacology is the science that deals with drugs. The word pharmacology is derived from two Greek words—*pharmacon* meaning 'an active principle' and *logos* meaning 'a discourse or treatise.' Pharmacology, in its broad definition, covers the physical and chemical properties, biochemical and physiological effects; mechanisms of actions; i.e., absorption, distribution, metabolism or biotransformation and excretion; and therapeutic uses of drugs. Pharmacology actually includes pharmacy, toxicology, chemotherapy, therapeutics, posology, etc. Pharmacology is concerned with the effect of drugs on living animals, organs or tissues. Clinical pharmacology applies pharmacological principles to the study of the effects and actions of drugs on humans.

The development of modern pharmacology as a science is fairly recent and probably began taking shape after the introduction of experimental procedures in animals by Francois Magendie (1783–1855) and Claude Bernard (1813–1878). Till then, the treatment of diseases was empirical, based on a combination of guess-work and experience. The spectacular developments in physiology, biochemistry, organic chemistry and molecular biology have greatly accelerated the advances in pharmacology. For the rational treatment of diseases, the knowledge of the mode of action of a drug, its effects on various body-systems and probable adverse effects, is important. The object of pharmacology, therefore, is mainly to provide such scientific data on both animals and humans, and this forms the basis of rational therapeutics.

1.4.2 Pharmacy

Pharmacy deals with the study of formulations of drugs. It is also concerned with the standardization of drugs. The mission of pharmacy is to serve the society with utmost professional responsibility in the appropriate use of medications, devices, and services, to achieve optimal therapeutic outcomes. Pharmacy includes the cultivation of medicinal plants, and the synthesis of compounds, along with chemical analysis.

Pharmacy concerns itself with the study that results in the discovery, development, and use of medications and medical information in the care of patients. It covers the clinical, scientific, economic and educational aspects of the medical profession and its communication to others in the health-care system. Further, pharmacy should ensure the maximum safety, cost-effectiveness and compliance by the patient.

1.4.3 Molecular pharmacology

The study of the action of drugs at the molecular level is known as molecular pharmacology. It includes the drug-receptor interactions, the affinity and efficacy of the drug molecules, and the structure-activity relationships. It also deals with the pharmacokinetics of the drug molecule, which takes care of the absorption, distribution in the body, metabolism, and elimination.

1.4.4 Medicinal chemistry

Medicinal chemistry is the science that deals with the discovery or design of new therapeutic chemicals and their development into useful medicines. It involves the synthesis of new compounds, evaluation of their biological activity, and a study of their interactions with receptors. It is also concerned with the determination of absorption and distribution properties, and studies of the metabolic transformations of drugs.

An understanding of the cause of a particular disease or illness can provide the basis for the development of drugs which are effective against it. Medicinal chemistry applies the principles of Chemistry and Biology to the creation and development of knowledge, leading to the development of new therapeutic agents for the benefit of mankind. The medicinal chemist must have a sound grounding in Biology, Biochemistry, Microbiology, and Pharmacology, besides being an efficient organic chemist. The

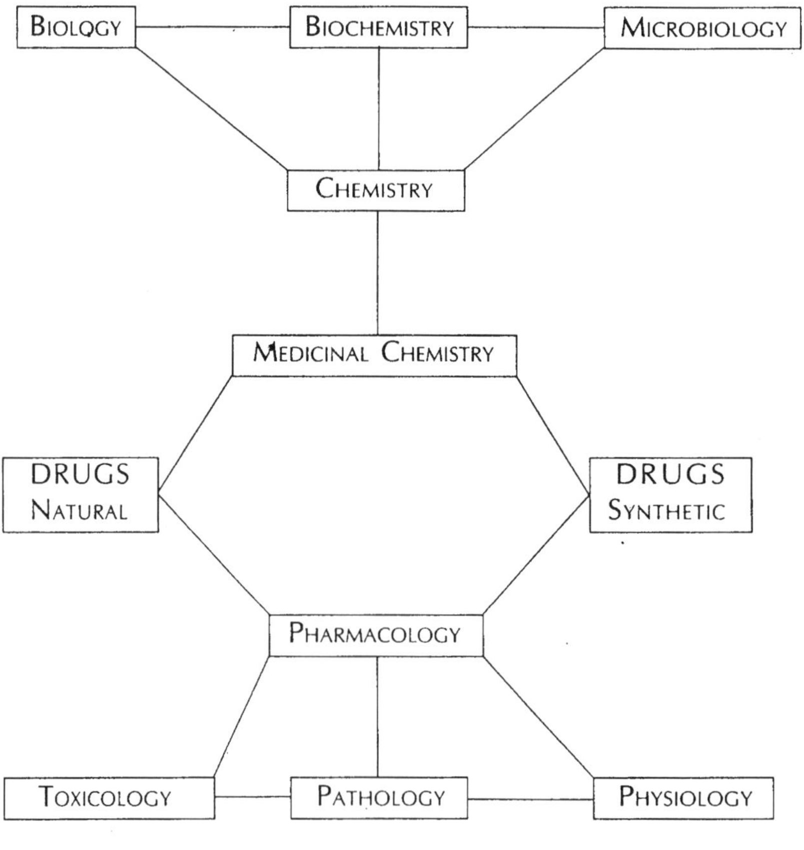

Fig. 1.1 *Interdisciplinary relationship between various related subjects and medicinal chemistry.*

interdisciplinary relationship between various related subjects and medicinal chemistry is indicated in a schematic diagram (Fig.1.1).

The relationship between medicinal chemistry and other disciplines provide us with the basis to develop suitable therapeutic agents.

1.4.5 Nomenclature

Medicinal compounds (drugs) normally have more than one name. Every proprietory drug (i.e., a drug which is sold under a trade name) has at least three names—a chemical name, a generic name, and a trade name (Fig. 1.2).

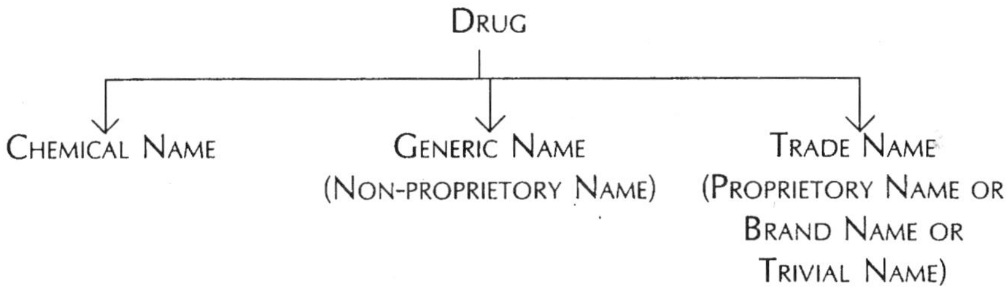

Fig. 1.2 *Nomenclature of drugs.*

When first discovered, a drug is given a chemical name on the basis of the IUPAC system. The chemical name describes the atomic or molecular structure of the drug. Usually, it is too complex and cumbersome for general use.

The generic name is assigned by an official body. In the USA, it is the FDA (Federal Drug Authority) that approves the drug for general prescription. The FDA assigns the generic name to the drug when it is first discovered and developed. Even if the same drug is later marketed by different manufacturers, it is known by the same generic name that was first approved of. The most important characteristic of a generic name is its uniqueness. (see page 142)

The trade name is chosen by the pharmaceutical company that manufactures it. The company tries to choose a unique name that is short and easy to remember. Trade names sometimes link the drug to its intended use or a particular characteristic of the drug. Trade names are also known as proprietory names or trivial names or brand names. A drug manufactured in one country and marketed in other countries may have different trade names in each country.

Individual drugs are almost always referred to by their generic names rather than by their trade or proprietory or brand names. Throughout this book, generic (non-proprietory) names have been used. However, because trade names are commonly used and may be more readily recognized, trade names are provided in brackets to several of the generic names mentioned in this book. Some of the generic names are listed along with their trade names (Table 1.1).

Table 1.1 *Generic and Trade Names*

Generic Name	Trade Name
Acetazolamide	Diomox
Alprazolam	Nitril, Quiet, Restyl, Alprax; Alzolam, Alzomax; Aten, Betanol
Amikacin	Amikin
Amlodipine	Amace
Amoxicillin	Amoxil, Novamax
Ampicillin	Omnipen, Polycillin
Analgin	Novalgin, Baralgan
Anisindione	Mirandon
Aspirin	Disprin, Micropyrin, Histagesic, Aspro, Equagesic, Anacin, Coldarin, Codopyrin
Atenolol	Sectral, Tenormin, Beta Card, Atelol, Aten, Betanol
Buspirone	Buscalm, Buspin
Benzythiazide	Exna
Bumetanide	Bumex, Burinex
Butamben	Butesin
Barbital	Veronal
Chlordiazepoxide	Librium
Cisapride	Syspride, Propulsid, Procisa
Carbamazepine	Tegretol
Captopril	Capoten, Capotril
Chlorothiazide	Diuril
Chloramphenicol	Chloromycetin
Chlorpheniramine	Teldrin
Chlorpromazine	Thorazine
Cimetidine	Tagamet
Ciprofloxacin	Cipro, Ciprobid, Alcipro, Ciplox, Ciprolet, Ciprodac
Clofibrate	Atromid-s
Diazepam	Calmpose, Valium
Diltiazem	Cardizen, Dilzen, Diltime
Dichlorphenamide	Daramide
Diphenhydramine	Benadryl
Desflurane	Suprane
Diclofenac	Voltaren
Enalapril	Vasotec, Envas; Vasopril, Invoril, En-Ace
Ethoxzolamide	Cardrase
Erythromycin	E-Mycin, Erythrocin
Felodipine	Plendil, Felogard
Furosemide	Lasix
Flumethiazide	Ademol
Fluoxetime	Prozac
Hydrochlorothiazide	Esidrix
Halothane	Fluothane
Haloperidol	Haldol
Isoflurane	Forane
Ibuprofen	Brufen
Isoproterenol	Isuprel
Lorazepam	Ativan, Larpose
Lidocaine	Dalcaine, Xylocaine
Lisinopril	Inras
LSD	Delysid
Lovastatin	Mevocor
Metoclopramide	Perinorm, Reglan, Maxeron-MPS
Metolazone	Diulo
Mephensin	Flamar, Paindex, Relaxyl, Cremalgin, Aristopyrin
Mebendazole	Vermox
Metronidazole	Flagyl
Methyl Dopa	Aldomet
Mexiletine	Mexitil
Nabumetone	Relafen
Nifedipine	Adalat, Calcigard, Procardia
Omeprazole	Prilosec, Omez
Paracetamol (Acetaminophen)	Crocin, Metacin, Calpal, Combiflam
Phenobarbital	Gardenal, Luminal
Phenothiazine	Emitil, Megatil, Siquil, Stemetil, Chlopramazine

(Continues...)

Table 1.1 (... *Contd.*)

Generic Name	Trade Name	Generic Name	Trade Name
Promethazine	Avomine, Phenergan	Ranitidine	Zantac, Ranitin
Procainamide	Pronestyl	Salbutamol	Ventolin
Pheniramine	Avil	Sulindac	Clinoril
Procaine	Novocaine	Terbutaline	Brethine
Propranolol	Inderal, Ciplar, Corbeta	Vinblastine	Velban
		Vincristine	Oncovin
Ramipril	Altace, Ramace	Warfarin	Coumadin

1.5 Pharmacokinetics

Pharmacokinetics is the study of Absorption, Distribution, Metabolism (biotransformation), and Excretion (ADME) of drugs. This study gives us information about the drug concentration in the blood and tissues at different time intervals (time-course of the drug) and will decide the dosage.

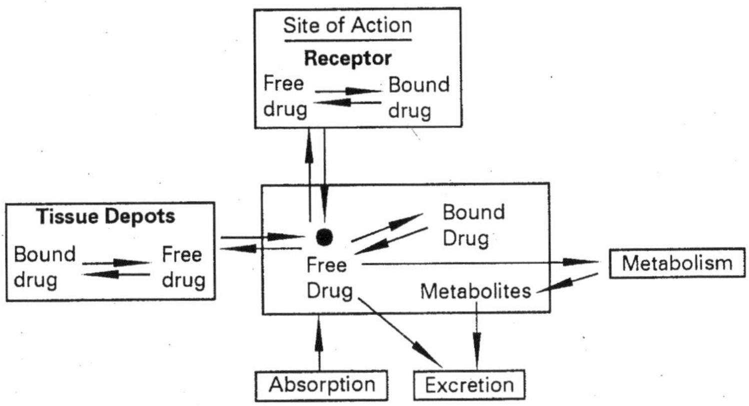

Fig. 1.3 *Schematic depiction of pharmacokinetics, i.e., the ADME factors.*

Digoxin (21) a cardiovascular drug, is effective in a once-daily dose; whereas aspirin (1), an analgesic drug, may need to be given 4 times a day. A dose of morphine is more effective if it is given intramuscularly, than if the same amount is taken orally. To know the reasons for these aspects, we have to study the pharmacokinetics of the drug. This deals with: (i) how drugs cross membranes (absorbed) to enter the body tissues, (ii) how they are distributed in the blood and other body tissues, (iii) how they are transformed (metabolized) to other compounds, and (iv) how they are eliminated (excreted) from the body (Fig. 1.3). It is necessary for the drugs to pass across cell membranes, which are essentially bilayers of lipid molecules.

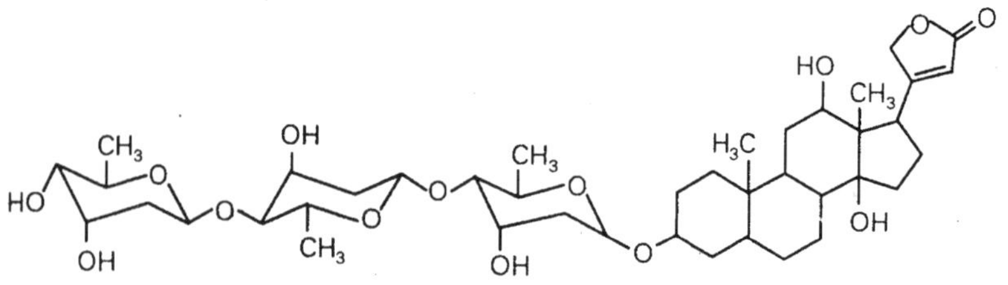

Digoxin (21)

1.5.1 Absorption

A drug is administered by: (i) oral (enteral), (ii) sublingual, (iii) intravenous (parenteral), (iv) intramuscular, (v) subcutaneous, (vi) rectal, (vii) pulmonary, and (viii) topical routes. When the drug is taken orally (the most common and desirable method of administration), it is absorbed mostly through the mucous membrane of the small intestine or the stomach (Fig. 1.4). The small intestine is the principal site for absorption, where most orally administered drugs enter the body. The stomach does not play a major role in absorbing drugs, because its area is much smaller than that of the small intestine, and also due to many other factors (the surface area of the small intestines is estimated to be that of a single's tennis court!). The degree to which a drug is lipid-soluble and ionized at intestinal pH also influences its absorption in the gut (intestine).

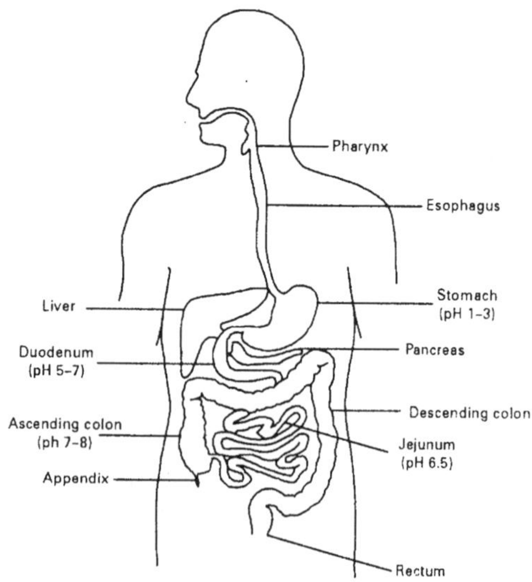

Fig. 1.4 *Anatomical diagram showing the digestive system including the locations involved in drug absorption, and their respective pHs.*

Once out of the gastrointestinal tract, it is carried via the bloodstream to the liver, where it is usually first metabolized. This drug metabolism by the liver enzymes is called the 'first-pass effect.' The first-pass effect can be avoided by changing the route of administration. The sublingual route (the drug placed under the tongue) bypasses the liver. After absorption through the buccal cavity, the drug enters the bloodstream directly. This route is used with nitroglycerin (22), a drug for *angina pectoris* (a heart condition). An intravenous (i.v.) injection introduces the drug directly into the systemic circulation, and is used when a rapid therapeutic response is desired. The effects are almost immediate when drugs are administered by this route, because the total blood circulation time in humans is about 15 seconds. Intramuscular (i.m.) injections are used when large volumes of drugs need to be administered or if slow absorption is desirable. A subcutaneous injection (s.c.) delivers the drug through the loose connective tissue of the subcutaneous layer of the skin. The rectal route, in the form of a solid like a suppository, or in solution as in an enema, leads to absorption through the colon mucosa. Ergotamine (23), a drug used for migraine headaches, is administered in this way. Another method of administration, particularly for gases or highly volatile drugs, such as anesthetics, is by pulmonary absorption through the respiratory tract. The asthma drug, isoproterenol (24) is metabolized in the intestines and liver, but administration of salbutamol (25) by aerosol inhalation is effective in getting the drug directly to the lungs. The topical application of the drug to the skin or mucous membrane is used for local effects.

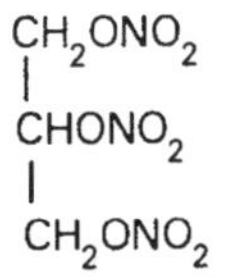

Nitroglycerin (22)
(Glonoin)

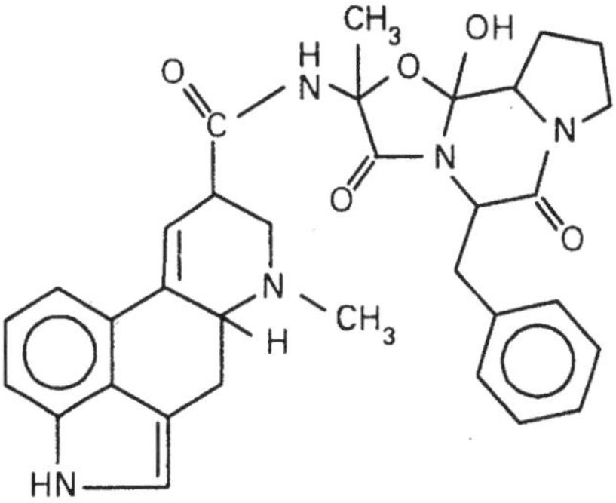

Ergotamine (23)

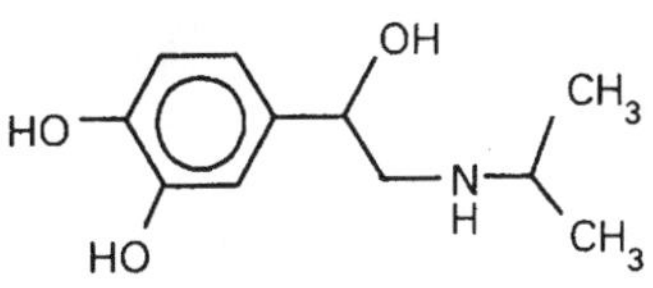

Isoproterenol (24)

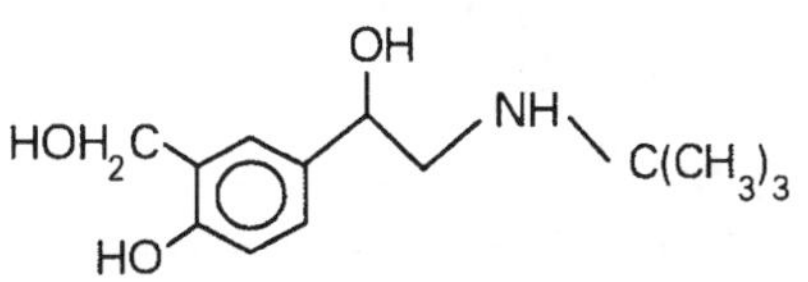

Salbutamol (25)

1.5.2 Distribution

If a drug is required to act throughout the body or to reach an organ inaccessible to topical administration, it must be sent into the blood and into other body compartments. Most drugs distribute widely, some dissolve in plasma water, some bind to plasma proteins, and some to tissues. The distribution is often uneven, as the drugs may bind selectively to plasma or tissue proteins or be localized within particular organs. The site of localization of a drug is likely to influence its action. The pattern of distribution from the plasma to other body fluids and tissues is a characteristic of each and every drug that enters the circulation and it varies enormously between drugs. If a drug remains mostly in the plasma, its distribution volume will be small, and if it is present mainly in the tissues, its distribution volume will include most of the body, i.e., it will be large. Drugs may also concentrate selectively in a particular tissue because of specialized transport mechanisms, e.g., iodine in the thyroid.

1.5.3 Metabolism

The enzymatic biotransformation of drugs is known as drug metabolism. Since many drugs have structures similar to those of endogenous compounds, they may be metabolized by specific enzymes. Drugs are treated by the body as foreign substances and various body mechanisms try to defeat the chemical intruders and eliminate them from the body. Some highly water-soluble drugs can be eliminated unchanged by the kidney, but others must first undergo structural modification, usually by enzyme action. Metabolic processes change drugs in two major ways: (i) by reducing lipid solubility, i.e., making them more polar for water solubility, and (ii) by reducing or increasing biological activity. Metabolic reactions tend to make a drug molecule progressively more water-soluble and so favour its elimination in the urine. During the process of metabolism, various steps that take place may have the following effects:

(i) Conversion of a physiologically active drug to an inactive substance. This is the case with most drugs.

(ii) Conversion of a physiologically active drug to another active substance.

E.g.1 Chloroquine $\longrightarrow$ Hydroxy chloroquine
E.g.2 Diazepam $\longrightarrow$ Oxazepam
E.g.3 Amitriptyline $\longrightarrow$ Nortriptyline

(iii) Conversion of a pharmacologically inactive substance to an active drug, i.e., a prodrug. A drug which is inactive when administered but utilizes the metabolic enzymes to convert itself into an active form, is known as a prodrug. The prodrug by itself has no drug property.

E.g. 1 Prontosil → Sulfanilamide
E.g. 2 L-Dopa → Dopamine
E.g. 3 Talampicillin → Ampicillin

A number of tissues, including the kidney, gut mucosa (gastrointestinal tract), lung and skin metabolize drugs, but the liver is by far the most important site, as many enzymes are present here. Drug metabolism reactions have been divided into two general categories termed as "Phase-I" and "Phase-II" reactions.

Phase I Phase I metabolism brings about a change in the drug molecule by oxidation, reduction or hydrolysis, and often introduces a reactive functional group into it. These reactions are catalyzed by enzymes.

For example

Oxidation – Propranolol is oxidized to hydroxy propranolol

Reduction – Nitrofurazone is reduced to 5–hydroxylamino derivative.

Hydrolysis – $COOCH_3$ gr is hydrolyzed to –COOH in the case of Cocaine (5).

Phase II In Phase II conjugating enzymes catalyze the attachment of small polar endogenous molecules such as glucuronic acid, sulphate, and amino acids to drugs or, more often, to metabolites of Phase-I enzymes. This further deactivates the drug and produces highly water-soluble metabolites that are readily excreted in the urine or in the bile.

1.5.4 Excretion

Drugs are eliminated from the body either unchanged or as metabolites. Generally, the more polar drugs are excreted readily. The less polar, lipid-soluble drugs, however, are not readily eliminated until they are metabolized to more polar, less lipid-soluble compounds. The kidney is the most important organ for drug excretion in the form of urine. Drugs excreted in the faeces are derived either from unabsorbed, orally-injested drugs or from metabolites excreted in the bile. Pulmonary excretion is of importance mainly for the elimination of anesthetic gases and vapours.

1.6 Pharmacodynamics

Broadly, the action of any drug involves two stages: (i) the journey of the drug molecule from its point of entry into the body (enterally, parentally, etc.) to the site of action (pharmacokinetics, i.e., ADME) and (ii) the interaction of the drug with the specific biological macromolecule of the human body (such as proteins or DNA), or the biological macromolecules (such as proteins or DNA) of the bacteria, in the case of bacterial infections (pharmacodynamics). The biological macromolecule in the human body or bacteria or virus with which the drugs bind, leading to the drug action, is called a **receptor**. These receptors are the targets for the drugs. Receptors are drug-recognition and drug-binding sites in the cells of the human body, tumour cells or bacteria. Receptors are located in different tissues of the body, e.g., CNS, lungs, gastric cells, and so on.

1.6.1 Receptors

Pharmacodynamics deals with the interaction of the drug with the receptor. This includes: (1) the recognition of the drug molecule by the receptor; (2) the binding of the drug with the receptor; generally by H-bonding or ionic bonding or van der Waals forces involving the functional groups of the drug and the functional groups of the receptor, and (3) translating the drug-receptor binding into a biological response (drug action). This entire series of action put together is known as **pharmacodynamics**.

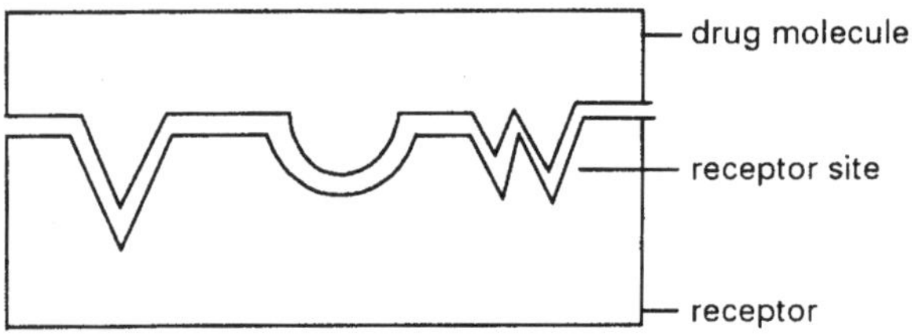

Fig. 1.5 *Lock and key model of the drug-receptor interaction.*

Paul Ehrlich, a noted microbiologist, is credited with coining the term 'receptor'. He observed that various organic compounds appeared to produce their antimicrobial effects with a high degree of selectivity. This led him to speculate that drugs produced their effects via binding to a biological substance, a receptor. Ehrlich considered that the interaction of the drug with the receptor was analogous to a **lock and key,** i.e., a specific molecular structure of the drug can interact to fit and bind with only one kind of receptor molecule (Fig. 1.5). The chemical functional groups of the receptor bind with the complimentary functional groups of the drug molecule (Fig. 1.6). The figure illustrates the antihypertensive drug, captopril, binding at the ACE receptor. One can observe H-bonding, ionic bonding, and ion-dipole bonding between the drug and the receptor. The site or spaces in the receptor molecule containing the functional groups that aid in binding to the drug is called the **receptor site**.

The receptors, which are chemically macromolecules, are mainly of two types: (i) protein receptors, and (ii) DNA receptors (Fig.1.7). The majority of receptors are proteins. A protein is a macromolecule (high molecular weight) and is built up of about 200–300 amino acid units. Proteins control and or catalyze all the cellular reactions and are responsible for all the cell functions. Many drugs are targeted to these protein receptors, to control or alter the cellular functions. DNA controls the replication of the cells. In the case of tumour (cancer), the cell multiplies more rapidly than the normal cells. Drugs can be targeted to the tumour cell DNA, (now called a receptor) which, by binding to it, can prevent the DNA replication and thereby control the tumour cell proliferation.

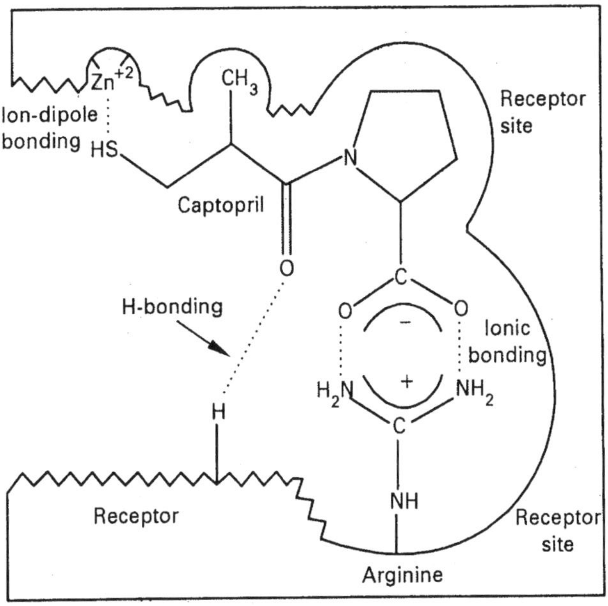

Fig. 1.6 *Captopril binding at the receptor, the Angiotensin Converting Enzyme (ACE).*

Receptors

- Protein Receptors (cellular reactions)
  - Non-catalytic H_1,H_2; β_1,β_2 receptors produce specific cellular activity (biological action), e.g.: salbutamol cimetidine
  - Catalytic receptors (enzymes) transform substrate into product (endogenous chemical into metabolites) enzyme inhibitors, e.g.: captopril, aspirin
- DNA Receptors (prevent replication)
  - Tumour cell DNA (in humans), e.g.: ethidium bromide, daunomycin, adriamycin
  - DNA of bacteria (in case of bacterial infection), e.g.: metronidazole

Fig. 1.7 *Classification of receptors.*

1.6.2 Protein receptors

In the human body, protein receptors are broadly classified into two classes: (i) non-catalytic protein receptors, and (ii) catalytic protein receptors (Fig. 1.7). In a normal situation, i.e., in the absence of the drug, the non-catalytic proteins (e.g: H_1 receptor, H_2 receptor, β_1-adrenergic receptor, β_2-adrenergic receptor) bind with an endogenous chemical (a chemical already present in the body), such as histamine and adrenaline, and produce specific cellular activity or functions.

Catalytic proteins are also known as enzymes. An enzyme, on the other hand, transforms an endogenous chemical (substrate) into another chemical (product). Enzymes catalytically produce several metabolites, which are responsible for the cellular functions.

Many diseases are due to the altered biochemistry of the cells, i.e., there is either a deficiency or excess of an endogenous chemical. In such a situation, the normal biological activity due to the non-catalytic or catalytic receptors is altered. A drug (exogenous chemical) is now needed to alter or regulate the specific biochemical reaction by interaction with the non-catalytic or catalytic receptors. The drugs are, therefore, targeted to these non-catalytic or catalytic receptors.

Non-catalytic protein receptors *(Example 1)* Adrenaline (26), an endogenous chemical, by binding to the β_1-adrenergic receptor produces bronchodilation. If there is less adrenaline in the body, it leads to symptoms of asthma. When salbutamol (25) is used as the drug, this drug binds with the β_1-adrenergic receptor to cause bronchodilation similar to that produced by adrenaline, as their chemical structures are similar. Salbutamol increases the overall bronchodilation. The bronchodilation is now due to both endogenous adrenaline and the drug salbutamol. Drugs like salbutamol, which bind with a receptor and produce a biological action similar to that of an endogenous chemical, are called **agonist** drugs.

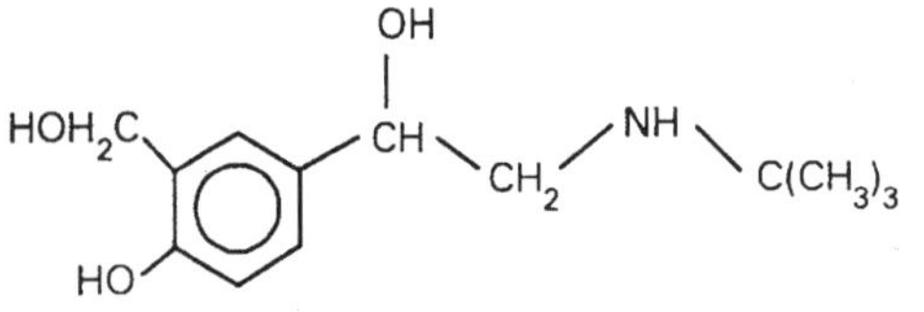

Salbutamol (25)

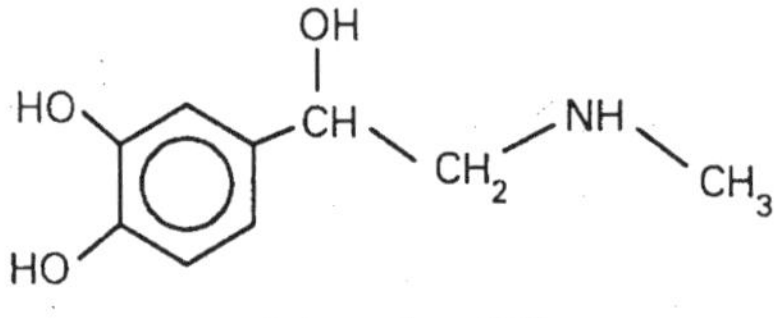

Adrenaline (26)

(Example 2) Histamine (27), on binding to the H_2 histamine receptor in the gastric cells, leads to the production of HCl which is necessary for the digestion of food. In people who suffer from tension, worry, etc., there is an excess production of HCl as more histamine is released in the gastric cells. Drugs like cimetidine (28) or ranitidine (29), whose chemical structure is not very similar to histamine, occupy and bind with the receptor

site on H_2 receptors and prevent the excessive production of HCl. So, there is now a competition between the histamine and cimetidine for the same H_2 receptor. The histamine-bound H_2 receptor as usual produces HCl, while the cimitidine-bound H_2 receptor cannot produce any HCl. Drugs like cimitidine which can only bind and block a receptor but do not produce any biological action, are known as **antagonists** or **blockers.**

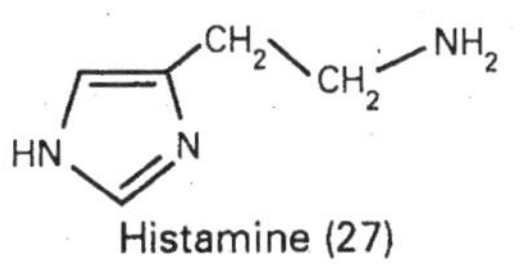

Histamine (27)

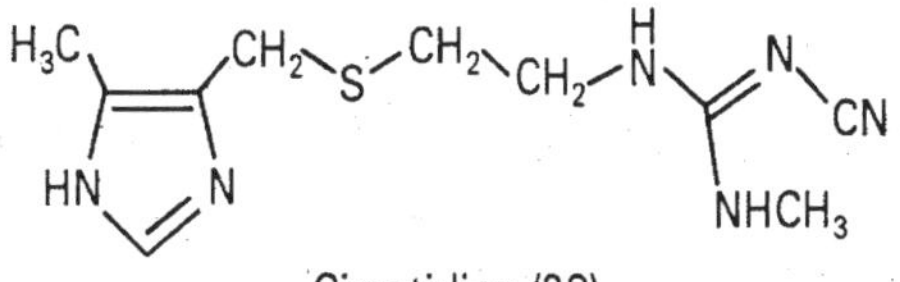

Cimetidine (28)

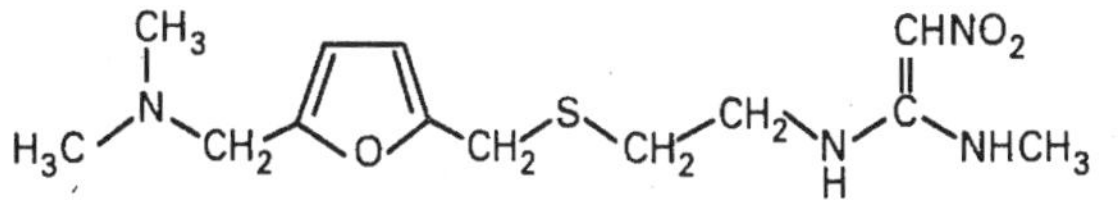

Ranitidine (29)

It should be clear by now that there are two aspects of drug-receptor interactions. They are: (i) the tendency of drug molecule to bind to the surface of the receptor, called the 'affinity' of the drug, and (ii) the ability of the drug-receptor-complex to initiate a biological response, which is called 'efficacy' or 'intrinsic activity'. The pharmacological activity depends on the rate of association and dissociation of the drug with the receptor. In general, while antagonists bind tightly to a receptor (great affinity), and are devoid of biological activity (no efficacy or intrinsic activity) (Fig.1.8b), agonists will have both affinity and efficacy (Fig.1.8a). In the case of agonists, the rate of both association and dissociation with the receptor would be quick (the latter quicker than the former). The rate of association of an antagonist with the receptor would be quick, but the dissociation would be slow.

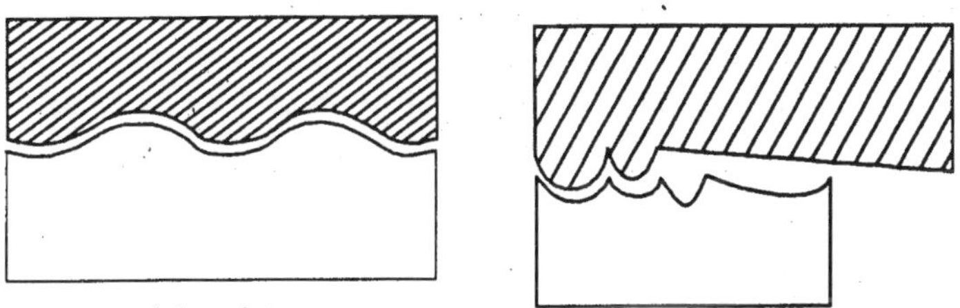

Agonist drug-receptor complex

(a)

Antagonist drug-receptor complex

(b)

Fig. 1.8 a & b *An agonist and antagonist drug-receptor complex.*

Catalytic Receptors *(Example 1)* An endogenous **chemical angiotensin-I,** a decapeptide, binds with the enzyme ACE (**Angiotensin Converting Enzyme**) and is transformed into an octapeptide, called **angiotensin-II, (Fig. 1.9)** mainly in the lungs, kidneys and blood vessels. This angiotensin-II is responsible for the increase in blood pressure by vasoconstriction. In persons with hypertension, due to stress, tension, etc., there is an increased production of angiotension-II by the ACE. Therefore, the person develops high blood pressure. Drugs like captopril (13), and enalapril (30), bind with the receptor site of ACE and block it. That is, there is a competition between angiotensin-I molecules and captopril molecules for the receptor site of ACE. As usual, the binding of angiotensin-I with ACE produces angiotensin-II which produces the blood pressure. But, captopril binding to ACE does not produce angiotensin-II. Therefore, overall, the blood pressure is lower now. The captopril drug molecules inhibit the ACE normal function. Drugs like captopril which block the enzyme and prevent its normal catalytic action, are known as **enzyme inhibitors**.

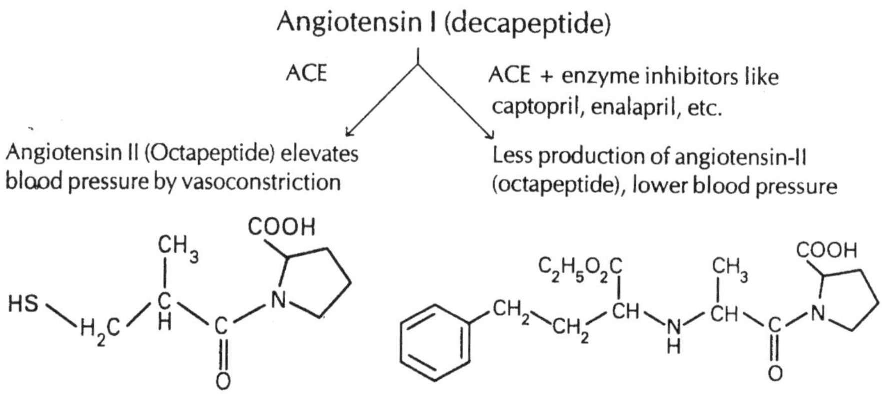

Captopril (13)

Enalapril (30)

Fig. 1.9 *Angiotensin-II production*

(Example 2) At the site of an injury, inflammation, infection, etc., the enzyme prostaglandin synthase (PGS) assists in the synthesis of prostaglandins. These prostaglandins are responsible for the pain and fever. Drugs like aspirin bind with prostaglandin synthase and block it, and prevent the production of prostaglandins. This results in anti-inflammatory, analgesic and antipyretic action. Aspirin is the inhibitor of the enzyme prostaglandin synthase (Fig. 1.10).

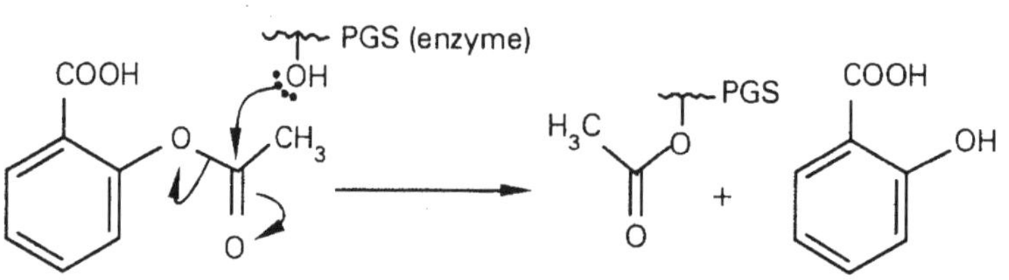

(1)

Salicylic acid

Fig. 1.10 *Mechanism for inactivation of prostaglandin synthase (PGS) by aspirin.*

1.6.3 DNA as receptors

(Example 1) In the case of bacterial infections, the drugs are targeted to the proteins or DNA of he bacteria present inside the human body. Penicillin is targeted to the bacterial enzyme *Peptidoglycan transpeptidase*. This enzyme, which controls the bacterial cell-wall synthesis, is inhibited, leading to the death of the bacteria. Dysentery, whose symptoms include diarrhoea, is caused due to bacterial infections. Metronidazole (31), a drug to cure dysentery, is targeted at the DNA of the bacteria. This drug breaks the DNA strands, causing bactericidal action.

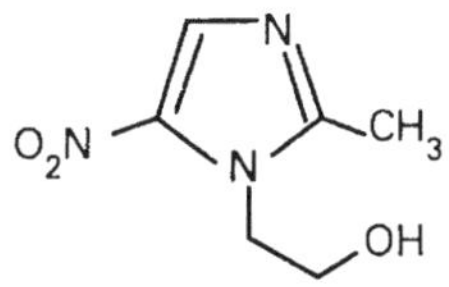

Metronidazole (31)

(Example 2) Drugs such as ethidium bromide (32), daunomycin and adriamycin are targeted at the DNA of the tumour cells. This drug molecule is inserted (intercalated) between the double helix of the DNA and thereby prevents its replication. This controls tumour growth.

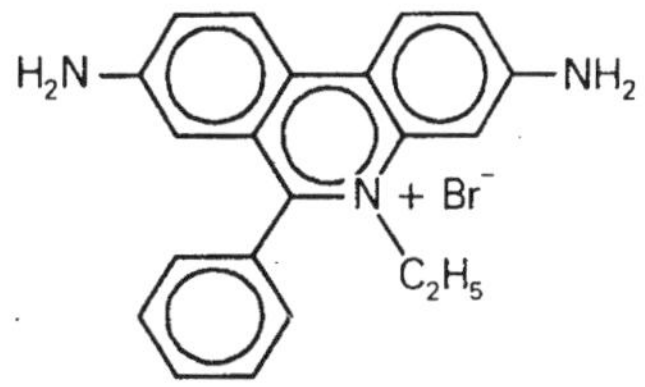

Ethidium bromide (32)

1.7 *Metabolites and antimetabolites*

1.7.1 Metabolites

Endogenous chemicals (chemical already present in the human body) as well as drugs are acted upon by a variety of enzymes to give transformed products. These enzyme-mediated transformation products are called metabolites. Metabolites are of two types:

(i) metabolites produced in the living cells and are useful for the cell functions.

(ii) metabolites produced from the drugs when they are acted upon by enzymes.

These drug metabolites have more, equal or less activity than the original drug. In short, the degraded products of drugs generated *in vivo* are called drug metabolites. In the process of drug discovery, the metabolism of the drug is thoroughly investigated. This involves the isolation and screening of the drug metabolites, in order to determine whether the activity observed is due to the drug or its metabolite. The following four examples illustrate the drug metabolites.

(Example 1) The anti-inflammatory drug, phenylbutazone (butazolidine) (8) is converted in the body into its metabolite oxyphenbutazone (33). The metabolite has one new hydroxyl group, which is introduced by the enzymatic transformation.

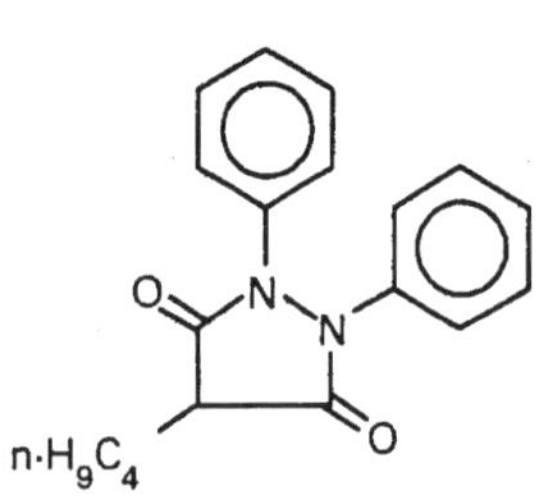

Phenylbutazone (8)
(Butazolidin)

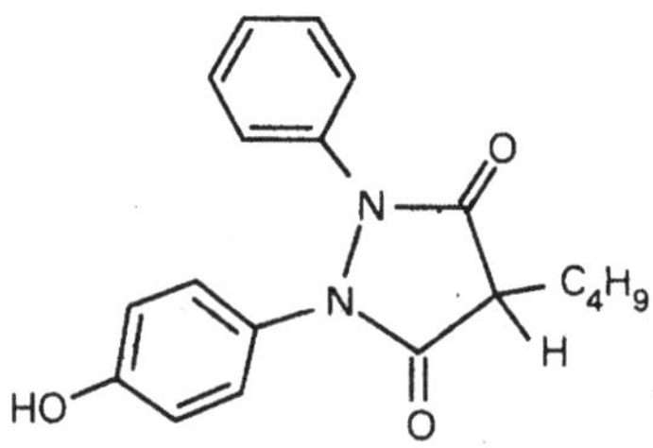

Oxyphenbutazone
(tandearil) (33)
Metabolite of phenylbutazone

(Example 2) Librium (34), a hypnotic/sedative drug, is metabolized in the body into demoxepam (35) and oxazepam (36). These two metabolites (Fig. 1.11) have a similar action to librium and, therefore, are also marketed as sedative drugs.

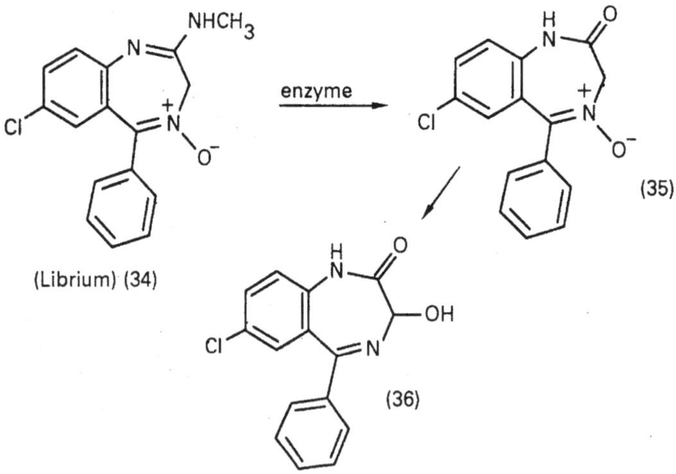

(Librium) (34)

(35)

(36)

Fig. 1.11 *Metabolites of librium.*

(Example 3) Some of the commonly used drugs are given in their prodrug forms. Prontosil (16) is an example of a prodrug that requires metabolic activation to be effective. Prontosil was found to have no activity against bacteria *in vitro*, but high activity *in vivo*. Trefouel and co-workers

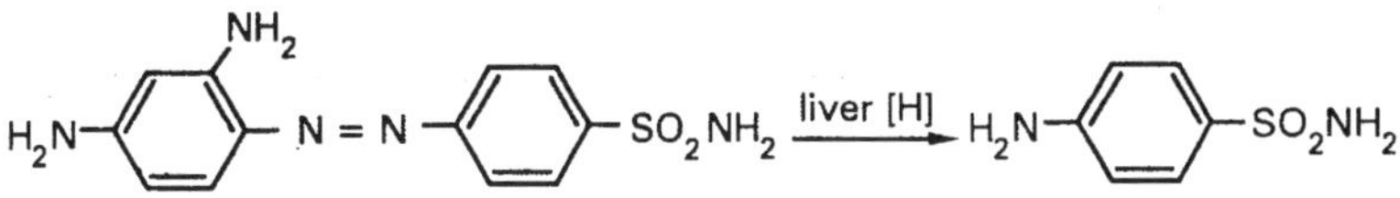

Prontosil (16) Sulphanilamide (17)

Fig. 1.12 *Metabolic transformation of prontosil to sulphanilamide.*

found that if a reducing agent was added to prontosil, it was effective *in vitro*. They suggested that the reason for the lack of *in vitro* activity, but high *in vivo* activity was that prontosil was metabolized to the active antibacterial agent, sulphanilamide (17). This metabolic transformation involves an enzymatic reduction (Fig. 1.12).

(Example 4) In the anti-inflammatory drug 'sulindac' (37), it is not the active agent but its metabolite (38) which is responsible for the activity. Sulindac is a prodrug and is used for rheumatoid arthritis, osteoarthritis and ankylosing spondolytis.

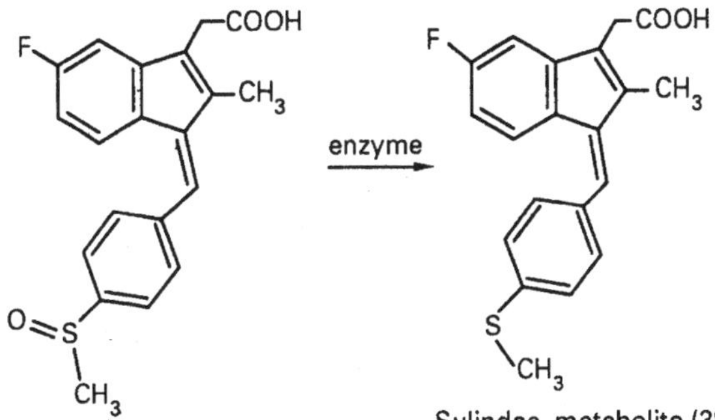

Sulindac (37) Sulindac metabolite (38)

1.7.2 Antimetabolites

Antimetabolites are drugs that mimic the natural substrate (metabolite) of an enzyme. The enzyme involved in a specific biochemical or metabolic pathway is thus inhibited. That is, a metabolite-like drug molecule is incorporated into the endogenous compound. For this reason, further biochemical functions of this drug-incorporated endogenous compound is prevented or disturbed.

(*Example 1:* Sulfa drugs) In bacteria, the endogenous compound dihydropteridine (39) reacts with Adenosine triphosphate (ATP), and accepts two phosphate groups to transform into dihydrophosphate. In this process, ATP is converted into adenosine monophosphate (AMP) by releasing the necessary two phosphate groups. The dihydropteridine diphosphate (40) combines with the endogenous substrate, or metabolite, p-amino benzoic acid (PABA) (41), by the action of an enzyme, *Dihydropteroate synthetase*, to give dihydropteroic acid (42). This dihydropteroic acid is converted into dihydrofolic acid (DHFA), which is further transformed into tetrahydrofolic acid (THFA). This THFA is needed for the purine synthesis which, in turn, is necessary for the bacterial DNA synthesis (Scheme 1). This is the normal process in bacteria (in the absence of a drug).

Sulfamethoxazole (43), a sulfa drug which has similar structural features as the essential metabolite of bacteria, the PABA, is used to treat bacterial infections. The bacterial enzyme *Dihydropterate synthetase* now uses sulfamethoxazole (43) as the substrate, mistaking it to be PABA, in the

SCHEME 1: Normal biochemical reaction in the bacteria

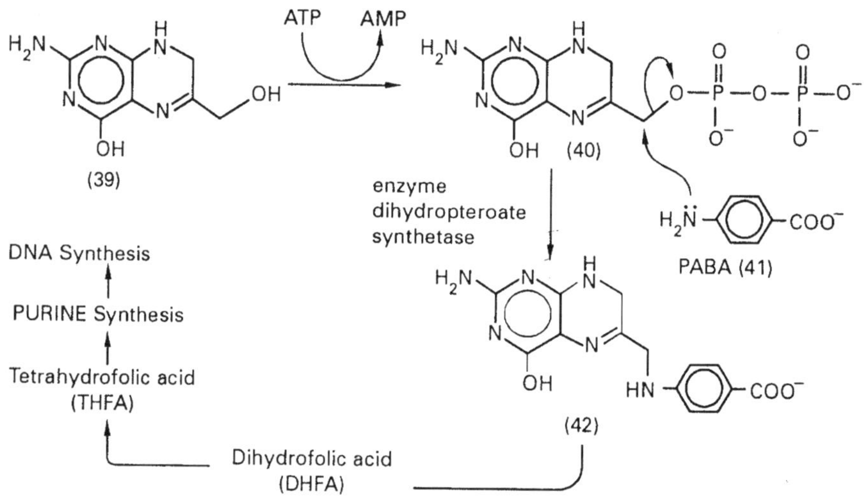

SCHEME 2: Biochemical reaction in the presence of an antimetabolite drug in bacteria

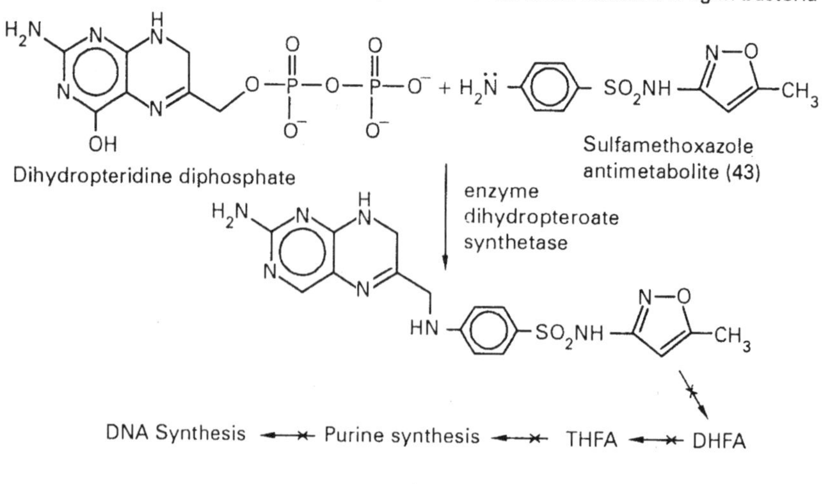

synthesis of dihydropteroic acid. The resultant product is not dihydropteroic acid but a biochemically wrong compound, as it contains the sulfamethoxazole moiety (Scheme 2). For this reason it cannot form DHFA and THFA and, therefore, cannot help in the purine synthesis or subsequent bacterial DNA synthesis. Hence, bacteria cannot multiply (bacteriostatic). Sulfamethoxazole is the antimetabolite.

Similarly, sulphanilamide (17) is also an antimetabolite as it is structurally similar to that of PABA (41).

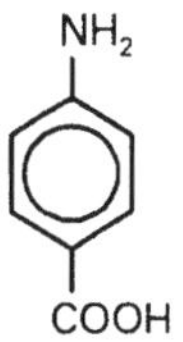

PABA (41)

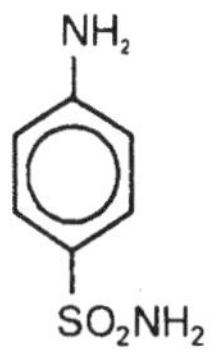

Sulphanilamide (17)

(Example 2) Purines, adenine, guanine, pyrimidines cytosine, and thymine are the essential substrates (metabolites) in the DNA biosynthesis. The DNA biosynthesis is similar in normal cells and tumour cells. However, in the tumour cells there is an elevated requirement of purines and pyrimidines. 5-fluorouracil (44) and its 2-deoxy-ribonucleoside (45) are the antimetabolite type of anti-tumour drugs. They are structurally similar to the natural metabolites, cytosine and cytidine and therefore, during DNA biosynthesis, get incorporated into the growing DNA strand. The enzymes involved in the DNA synthesis are unable to discriminate between uracil (46) and the structurally similar 5-fluorouracil (44). The DNA obtained now contains 5-fluorouracil incorporated in it and, therefore, this 'wrong' DNA cannot replicate or perform its normal function. The tumour cell growth (proliferation) is thus controlled.

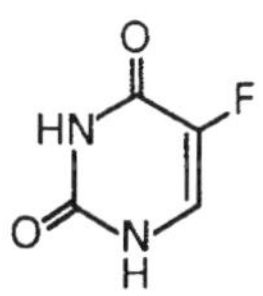

5-fluorouracil (44)

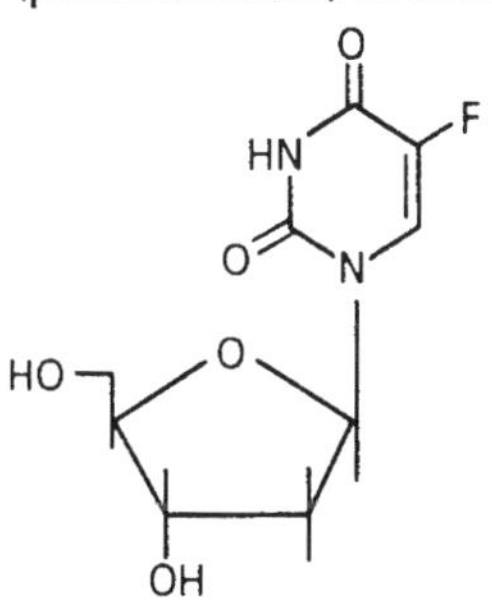

2-deoxy-ribonucleoside (45)

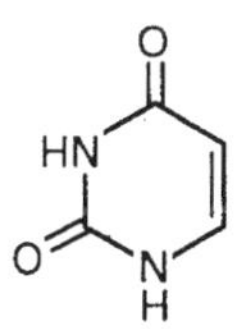

Uracil (46)

Thus, antimetabolites are the structural analogs of a metabolite that can bind to the enzyme/receptor sites and inhibit or block cellular growth, but do not undergo the normal chemical reactions of the metabolite or produce the usual physiological response.

1.8 Pharmacophore

The parts of the drug molecule that interact with the receptor and are responsible for biological activity are known as the pharmacophore of the compound. Any structural alterations of the pharmacophore from the molecule of a drug either lessens or totally destroys its medicinal value.

Ibuprofen (11), naproxen (47) and ketoprofen (48) are anti-inflammatory drugs differing slightly in their potency and duration of action. The common structural feature in all the three anti-inflammatory drugs is aryl methylacetic acid (49).

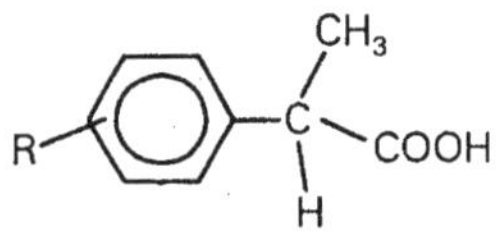

Arylmethylacetic acid (49)

This molecular skeleton (49) is responsible for the similar biological activity of all these drugs, as it binds at the specific receptor responsible for control of pain or inflammation. The molecular fragment (shown with dotted lines) which binds with the receptor and is responsible for its biological action, is called the pharmacophore of the drug. Therefore, the pharmacophore is related to the pharmacodynamics of the drug. The other part of the drug molecule is commonly called the non-pharmacophore of the drug. The non-pharmacophore mostly decides the pharmacokinetics of the drug, i.e., the rate of drug absorption, duration of action and drug metabolism. Changes in the molecular structure of the pharmacophore part lead to the loss of a specific drug property, while changes in the non-pharmacophore part may not change the drug properties.

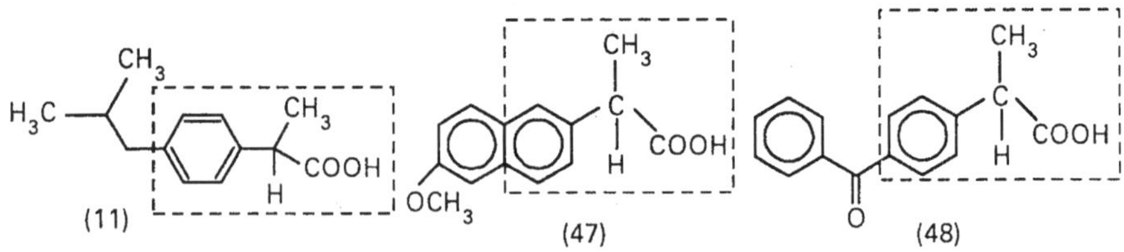

(11) (47) (48)

All anti-allergic drugs (also known as H_1 receptor antagonists) have the same pharmacophore as that of diphenhydramine (Benadryl) (50) and chlorpheniramine (51). In these two compounds, the common molecular skeleton responsible for the anti-allergic action is $(Ar)_2X–CH_2–CH_2–N(CH_3)_2$. This fragment of the drug molecule is the pharmacophore which binds with the H_1 histamine receptor and, thereby, blocks the allergy symptoms (rash, sneezing, asthma, etc.).

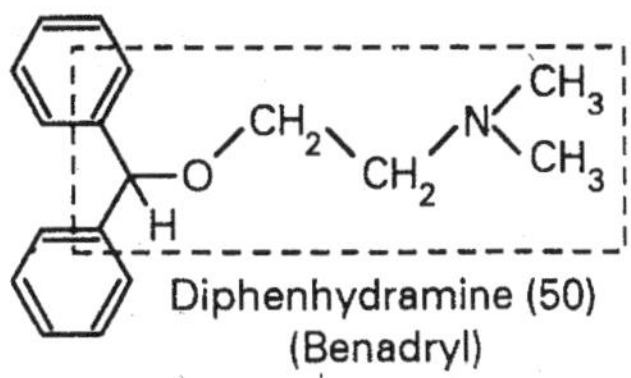

Diphenhydramine (50)
(Benadryl)

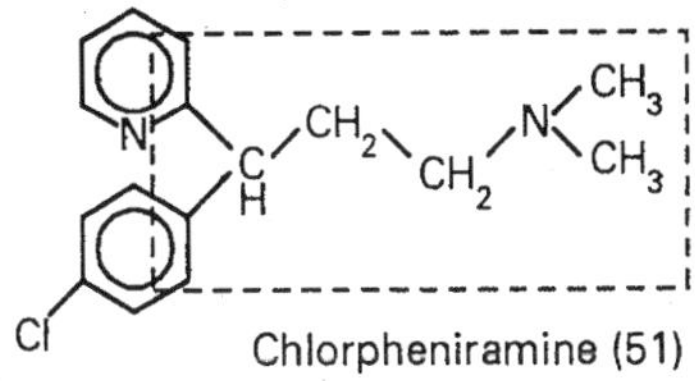

Chlorpheniramine (51)

1.9 Bacteria

Bacteria are the simplest microscopic, prokaryotic, unicellular organisms. They are highly adaptable and can survive extremes of temperature, atmospheric pressure and pH and are, therefore, found in all natural environments. They are very resistant and can withstand cold (−190°C) and heat (≈ 75°C). They are present everywhere—in water, air, soil, in all living organisms, animals and plants.

Size Bacteria are the minutest organisms. The smallest bacteria are about 0.1 micron, while the largest may be 60 × 6 microns.

Shape Bacteria occur in three main shapes: spherical, rod-like and spiral. The spherical ones are called cocci (singular-coccus). Cells may occur in pairs (diplococci), in groups of four (tetracocci), in bunches (staphylococci), chain-like (streptococci) or in a cubical arrangement (sarcinae). Rod-like bacteria are called bacilli (singular-bacillus). Mostly they occur singly, but are sometimes found in pairs (diplobacilli) or chains (streptobacilli). Spiral bacteria are called spirilla; short, incomplete spirals are called vibrios (comma-like) (Fig. 1.13).

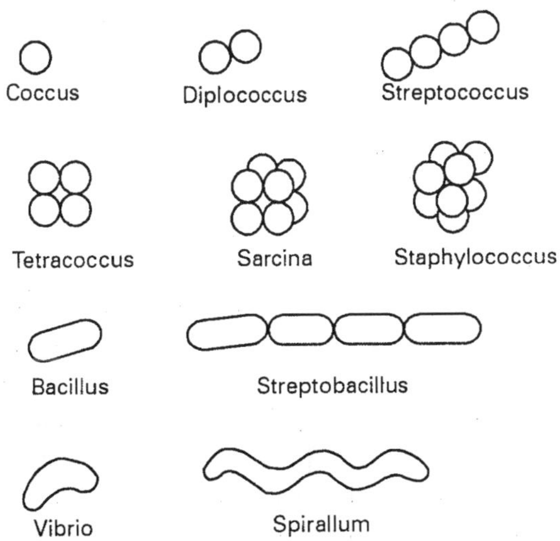

Fig. 1.13 *Shapes of bacteria.*

Anton Van Leuwenhock (1676) is credited with the discovery of bacteria. He found them first in rain-water, then in pond-water, and later in scum (material from his own teeth). After 200 years, it was Louis Pasteur in France and Robert Koch in Germany, who elaborated the work on bacteria and established that bacteria and other microbes could bring about chemical changes like fermentations, and are also the cause of many diseases in plants, animals and human beings. Pasteur's work indicated that bacteria and yeast were tiny chemical factories that could bring about important chemical changes. Emil von Behring, Koch's associate, was able to treat diphtheria successfully in 1890 by injecting a patient with antitoxin. Kohn (1882) also isolated the tuberculosis bacteria. During the golden age of microbiology (1860–1950), many workers discovered that the causal organisms of many human diseases are different bacteria and have also extracted many antibiotics from the same. Bacteria that cause some common human diseases are given in Table 1.2.

Table 1.2 *Common Human Diseases Caused by Bacteria*

Disease	Name of the Bacterium
Meningitis	*Nisseria meningitidis*
Pneumonia	*Diplococcus pneumoniae*
Typhoid	*Salmonella typhi*
Boils, Carbuncles	*Staphyloccus aureus*
Diphtheria	*Corynobacterium diptheriae*
Whooping cough (Pertusis)	*Bordetella pertusis*
Tetanus	*Clostridium tetani*
Botulism	*Clostridium botulinum*
Cholera	*Vibrio comma*
Syphilis	*Treponema pallidium*
Gonorrhoea	*Nisseria gonorrhoea*
Plague	*Pasteurella pestis*

1.9.1 Structure of a typical bacterial cell

A typical bacterial cell consists of a cell wall which gives shape to the cell (Fig. 1.14). Beneath the cell wall is the plasma membrane or cytoplasmic membrane which encloses the protoplasm. The plasma membrane is thin and semi-permeable. Chemically, it is lipoproteinous with small amounts of carbohydrates. The protoplasm consists of cytoplasm and a nuclear body. The bacterial nucleus has no nuclear membrane or nucleolus. The genetic material (genome) consists of a single molecule of double-stranded DNA arranged in the form of a circle.

Such a type of nucleus is called an 'incipient nucleus' and organisms possessing such a nucleus are called prokaryotes, in contrast to the definite nucleus present in eukaryotes.

The bacterial cytoplasm is a colloidal system. It consists of organelles like ribosomes, mesosomes, and vacuoles. Mitochondria and endoplasmic reticulum, which are essentially present in eukaryotes, are not found in bacteria (prokaryotes). Some bacteria are surrounded by a capsule. This capsule is secreted by the bacterial cell and is usually composed of polysaccharides. Though the capsule is not necessary for the survival of the bacteria, its presence is important in their disease-causing ability. For example, the non-capsulated laboratory strains of *Pneumococcus* (pneumonia-causing) are destroyed by host phagocytes and are non-infectious, whereas encapsulated strains avoid phagocytosis and hence are virulent (disease causing).

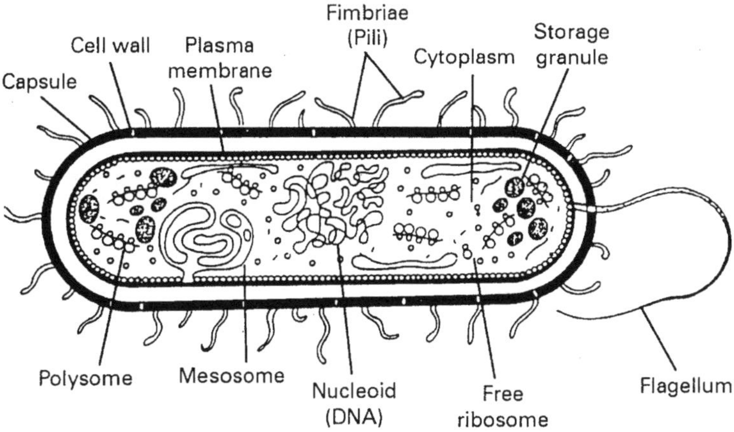

Fig. 1.14 *Structure of a bacterial cell.*

1.9.2 Gram stain

A Danish scholar, Christian Gram (1884), devised a staining procedure to differentiate between the two kinds of bacteria. Crystal violet solution is applied to the bacteria for 30 seconds. The bacteria are gently rinsed in clean water and iodine solution is applied for 30 seconds. Now, all the bacteria cells become violet. These stained bacteria cells are to be washed with 95% ethyl alcohol. The bacteria which retain the violet colour are called Gram-positive, and the others which lose the violet colour are called Gram-negative.

The basis of this differential stain lies in the chemistry of the bacterial cell walls, which causes certain bacteria to react differently.

Some bacteria are autotrophic (self-feeders) and others heterotrophic (feeding on others). Autotrophs are of two types: phototrophs, which use the energy drawn from the sunlight for preparation of food and chemotrophs, which depend upon inorganic chemicals for the synthesis of food. Heterotrophs also are of two types: parasites and saprophytes (Fig. 1.15).

While saprophytes live on dead and decaying organic matter, parasites survive on living organisms (i.e., on plants, animals and human beings) causing dreaded diseases. Respiration is the process of oxidation in which energy is released. In bacteria, respiration may be aerobic or anaerobic. The common method of multiplication is by binary fission: one cell divides into two cells of equal size. Bacterial reproduction is very rapid, with many species dividing once in every 20 minutes.

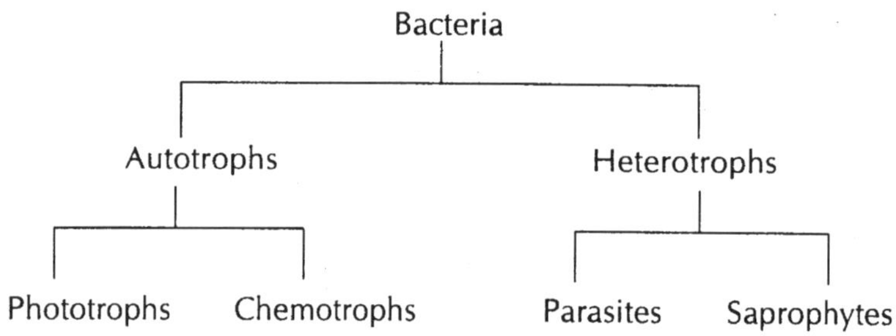

Fig. 1.15 *Classification of bacteria.*

1.9.3 Importance of bacteria

It is often said that bacteria are both friends and foes of mankind, as they display some useful activities as well as some harmful activities. The beneficial activities of bacteria are: (i) decomposition of waste matter serving as natural scavengers, (ii) helping some fungi in mineral cycling between the ecosystems, (iii) increasing the soil fertility by fixing free atmospheric nitrogen which green plants cannot do, (iv) some bacteria like *Escherichia coli* help in human digestion, (v) biological control of pests, (vi) many metabolic activities of commercial value like tanning of leather, and natural gas production, (vii) producing many industrial chemicals, organic acids, and enzymes, (viii) production of antibiotics; e.g., streptomycin, terramycin, chloromycin, erythromycin, neomycin, etc. are prepared from bacteria, and (ix) bacteria are now being used in recombinant DNA technology.

Their harmful activities include: (i) the causing of various diseases of plants, animals and humans, (ii) denitrification of the soil, (iii) spoilage of foodstuff, (iv) pollution of water and air, and (5) causing abortion in animals.

1.10 Fungi

Fungi are an eukaryotic, achlorophyllous (non-green), spore-bearing group of plants. Mycology is the science of fungi. From the seventeenth century onwards, work has been progressing in the field of mycology. Many fungi that cause diseases in plants and animals, and some useful fungi that produce antibiotics have been found and studied extensively. Fungi have been recognized as the causative agents of human disease earlier than bacteria. Various fields of study of fungi have developed now like Microbiology, Plant Pathology, Medical Mycology, and Industrial Mycology.

Fungi are highly diversified in their habitat; they may be aquatic (present in water) or terrestrial (soil). While some species are microscopic, some others are macroscopic, like mushrooms, puffballs, bracket fungi, and cup-fungi. As fungi are invariably achlorophyllous, their mode of nutrition is heterotrophic (feeding on others). Heterotrophs are of two types: (i) Saprophytes which live on dead and decaying matter, and (ii) Parasites which live on other living organisms like plants and animals, including humans. They cause infectious diseases, some of which are very serious in nature. The pathogen (fungus) absorbs its food material readily from the host.

Importance of Fungi Fungi are useful as well as harmful to man.

The useful activities:

1. **Source of chemicals:** Fungi are a source of chemicals and are used in many industries to produce compounds like organic acids, alcohols, glycerol, lipids, enzymes, vitamins, and alkaloids.

Table 1.3 *Some Useful Antibiotics of Fungal Origin*

Antibiotics	Produced by	Active against
Penicillins	*Pencillium chrysogenum*	Gram +ve, and Gram -ve bacteria
Cephalosporins	*Acremonium spp.*	Gram +ve bacteria
Griseofulvin	*Pencillium griseofulvum*	Most fungi
Fusidic acid	*Fusidium coccineum*	Gram +ve bacteria

2. **Source of medicines:** About 770 antibiotics have been discovered from fungi, though only a few of them are commercially used. Some useful antibiotics of fungal origin are given in Table 1.3. Penicillin occupies an important place among the antibiotics isolated from fungi, as it is a very useful broad-spectrum antibiotic that has been used to save mankind from many dreaded diseases. In 1929, Alexander Flemming observed that a colony of *Pencillium notatum,* contaminating bacterial culture, inhibited bacterial growth. He called this antimicrobial principle

pencillium and used this to eliminate Gram +ve bacteria. The famous drug 'ergotin' which has long been used to induce uterine contractions is obtained from the fungus, *Claviceps purpuria*.

3. **Source of food:** A wide range of foods are obtained from fungi which are relatively more popular in western countries. Mushrooms, protein cakes (prepared by mixing yeast in cereal flours), fermented foods like tempeh, tapioca, and cheeses, are the some important food products of various fungi.
4. **Alcohol production:** Saccharomyces (commonly called yeast) is a unicellular fungus which is of great help in the brewing (preparation of malt and alcohol) industry.
5. **Biological assays:** Some fungi, like *Neurospora crassa and Asperigillus niger,* are used to assay drug potency and in the detection of some metals like Zn, Pb, Cu, Mn and Mb.
6. **Soil fertility:** Some soil-fungi secrete mucilaginous (sticky) substances which have soil binding properties. Some fungi have nitrogen-fixing capabilities.
7. **Decomposers:** Fungi help in the recycling of mineral nutrients between the soil and the atmosphere (through the decomposition of dead organic matter).
8. **Biological control of pests:** Some fungi are antagonistic to other fungi, like bacteria, nematodes, and insects, which arė serious pathogens.
9. **Biofertilizers:** Some fungi live in and on the roots of higher plants and help the plant in increased absorption of water and minerals. They are good examples of symbiosis and are called mycorrhizae (rhizine = root; myco = fungus: root fungus). Nowadays, they are considered as biofertilizers.

Table 1.4 *Common Human Diseases Caused by Fungi*

Disease	Principal Tissue Involved	Fungus
Dermatomycosis (ring worm)	Skin, hair, nails	*Epidermatophyton flocossum*
Aspergillosis	External ear, lungs, eye, brain	*Aspergillus* spp.
Blastomycosis	Lungs, skin, bone, testes	*Blastomyces dermatidis*
Candidiasis	Gastrointestinal and urogenital tracts, skin, mucosa	*Candida albicans*
Mucormycosis	Nasal mucosa, lungs, blood vessels, brain	*Rhizopus, Mucor, Absidia*
Sporotrichosis	Skin, joints, lungs	*Sporothrix schenckii*
Madura foot	Foot	*Nocardia* spp.

The harmful activities are

1. **Destruction of matter:** Deterioration of paper, textiles, leather, plastics, rubber, wool, painted surfaces, cable- wire insulations, photographic articles, etc., is caused by fungi.
2. **Mycotoxins:** Some fungi produce toxins that spoil food materials. Mycotoxins are secondary fungal metabolites which, when consumed by man and animals, cause a state of intoxication termed 'Mycotoxicosis.'
3. **Disease causing:** Fungal infections are extremely common in plants, animals, and human beings, and some of them are even fatal. Some of the common diseases caused by fungi in man are given in Table 1.4.

1.11 Viruses

Viruses are submicroscopic organisms that can infect the living cells. They are parasitic, multiply at the expense of the host's metabolic system, and are potentially pathogenic.

Viruses are among the smallest microorganisms, varying in size from 0.02 to 0.04 μm. They can be seen and identified with the help of an electron microscope. Viruses consist of a nucleic acid core that contains either deoxyribonucleic acid (DNA) or ribonucleic acid (RNA), which constitute the genetic material and provide a basis for classification of viruses. Fundamentally, viruses are classified into two main groups, namely DNA-containing viruses and RNA-containing viruses. The nucleic acid core is surrounded by a protein coat known as the capsid. The entire structure is called the nucleocapsid. The nucleocapsid may or may not be covered by another protein coat called the envelop. The arrangement of the coat proteins defines the overall shape of the viruses. Spheres, rods, filaments, bullets, rectangles, triangles and elongated tubes are some of

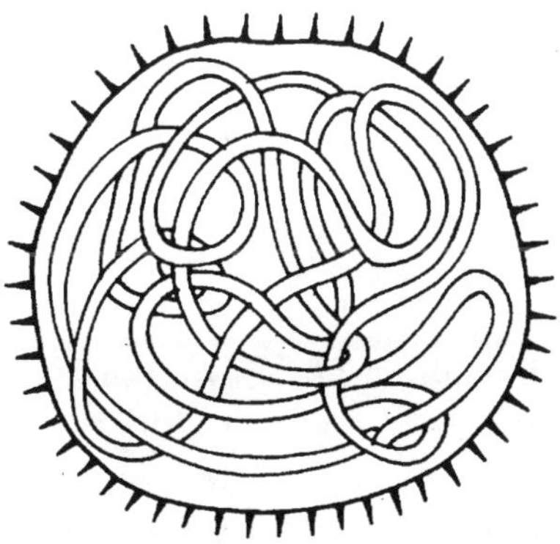

Mumps Virus

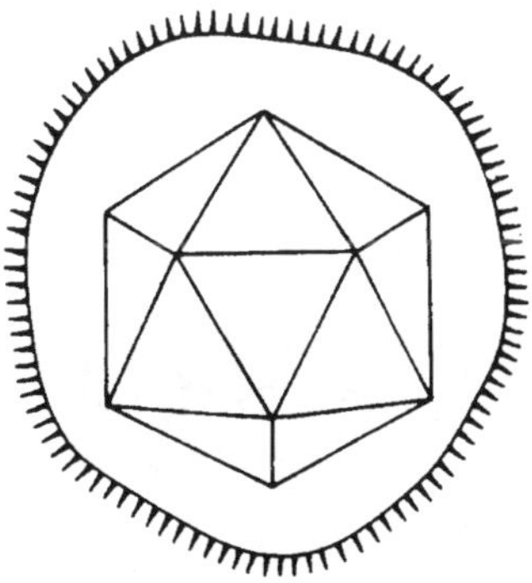

Herpes Virus

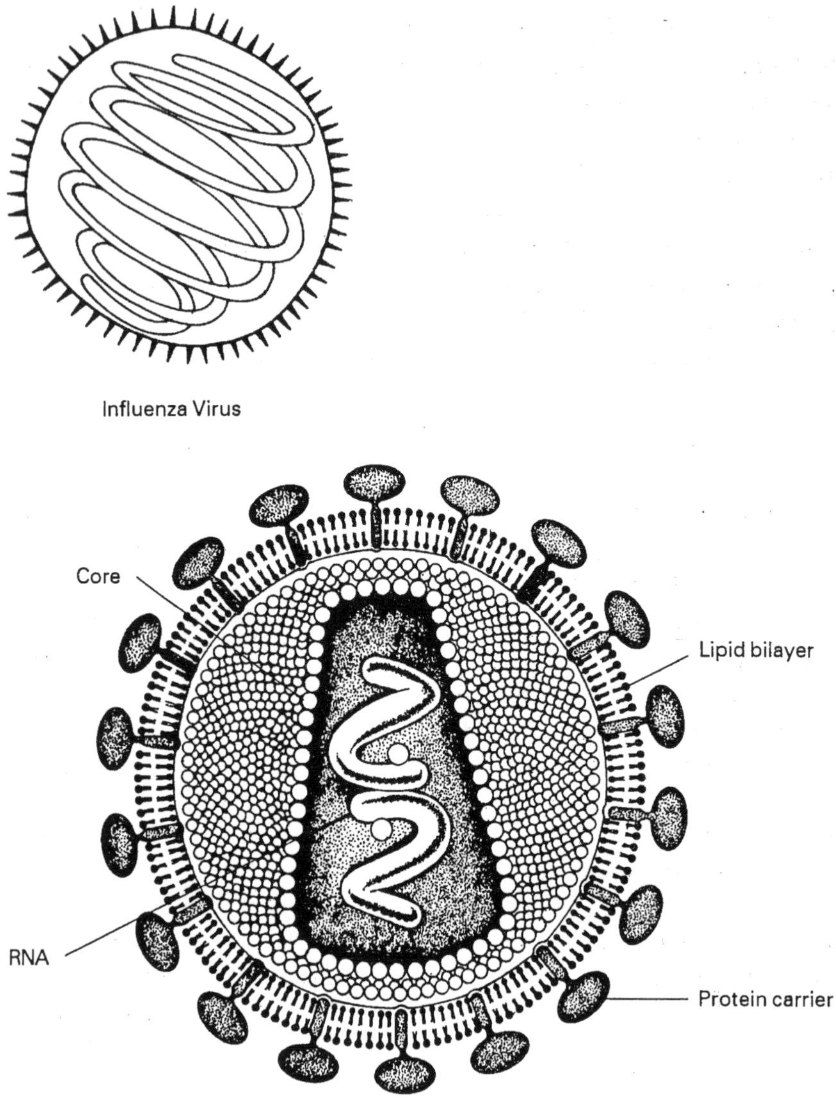

Fig. 1.16 *The structure of viruses.*

the shapes of viruses (Fig. 1.16). The complete infectious virus particle is called a 'virion'.

The major routes of transmission of viral infections in humans are through the respiratory, gastrointestinal and genital tract, the skin, urine, blood and placenta. Viral infections may occur through air, water, food, milk, or other sources. The nature of the protein coats of the virus and the absence or the presence of the envelope play an important role in the initial stages of viral infection. The reactive sites on the capsid or the envelope become attached to the receptor sites on the host cell. The penetration, uncoating and release of the virions in the host cell depends on the structural coat protein. This process influences the susceptibility of the virus to the actions of anti-viral agents. The diseases caused by viruses in animals and human beings are given in Table 1.5.

Table 1.5 *Viruses Infecting Animals and Human Beings*

Virus Group		Disease
DNA-containing viruses		
Adenovirus	–	Respiratory tract and eye infections (keratitis)
Herpes virus	–	Encephalitis, eye infections, skin diseases, genital infections, chickenpox
Papova virus	–	Animal and human warts, salivary gland (parotid) infection
Pox virus	–	smallpox, chickenpox, eczema
RNA-containing Viruses		
Arena virus	–	Lymphocytic choriomenengitis (LCM), hemorrhagic fever
Orthomyxo virus	–	Influenza
Paramyxo virus	–	Mumps, measles, para-influenza (pneumonia, bronchiolitis)
Picorna virus	–	Respiratory diseases, gastrointestinal diseases, poliomyelitis, aseptic meningitis
Reo virus	–	Mild respiratory and gastrointenstinal symptoms
Retro virus (Oncorna virus)	–	Leukemia, lymphoma in animals, human breast cancer, human T-cell leukemia, nasopharyngeal carcinoma, AIDS
Rhabdo virus	–	Rabies, encephalitis
Toga virus	–	German measles (Rubella), meningo-encephalitis, encephalitis, hepatitis, yellow fever

Viruses differ from bacteria in several respects. (i) Bacteria are cellular organisms while viruses are acellular. (ii) A virus can multiply only in living tissue, while outside it is an inert chemical. They can be crystallized outside; whereas, bacteria act as living organisms both outside and inside the living organism. (iii) All viruses are pathogenic, while only a few bacteria are pathogenic and several are useful. (iv) A virus does not possess its own mechanism for energy production and protein synthesis. (v) Viruses are not affected by antibiotics.

1.12 Mutations

The sudden, heritable change of a gene in an organism is known as mutation. It is a random, undirected variation caused by an alteration in the nucleotide sequence at some point in the DNA of the cell. It may be due to addition, deletion or substitution of one or more bases of DNA. All genes are susceptible to mutations, but not all mutations are expressed. Some mutations involve vital functions. Mutation is a natural event, taking place all the time at its particular frequency in all organisms. Most mutations, however, go unrecognized as the mutation may affect some minor function that may not be expressed. Mutation is significant when it involves a function which can be readily observed. For example, an *E. coli* mutant that loses its ability to ferment lactose can be readily detected. If a streptomycin-resistant mutant of the Tubercle Bacillus (TB) develops in a patient under- going drug treatment, it multiplies selectively and ultimately replaces the original drug-sensitive population of bacteria. But in a patient who is not undergoing treatment, the mutation confers no survival advantage and, therefore, preferential multiplication of the mutant does not occur.

The mutation may be spontaneous or induced and is inherited by the subsequent generations. This remains until a further mutation occurs. Each gene undergoes mutation with a fixed frequency. The mutation rates of individual genes in bacteria range from 10^{-2} to 10^{-10} per bacterium per division.

The molecular mechanism of mutation is that, during DNA replication, some 'error' creeps in. For instance, instead of thymine bonding with adenine it may, due to tautomerism, sometimes bond with guanine. The progeny copies this error (change). Though mutation occurs spontaneously, its frequency can be increased by several agents (mutagens) such as UV rays, alkylating agents, acridine dyes, 5-bromo-uracil, and 2-amino purine.

Spontaneous mutation takes place without apparent influence from outside the cell, while induced mutation is produced by a known agent outside the cell, e.g., UV radiation, X-rays, etc. Mutation may alter any gene and hence may modify any characteristic of the organism. The mutants may vary in properties such as nutritional requirement, biochemical reaction, antigenic structure, morphological features, colony form, drug susceptibility, virulence, host range, etc.

The practical importance of bacterial mutation lies mainly in the field of drug resistance and the development of live vaccines.

2 PHARMACODYNAMIC AGENTS

2.1 Classification of drugs–criteria

Drugs are generally categorized into two groups. They are: (i) based on their chemical structure and (ii) based on their therapeutic actions.

Chemical structure basis A similarity in functional groups or ring systems is the basis of this category. Acids, alcohols, phenols, ethers, esters, nitro compounds, amino compounds, amides, amino alcohols, amino ethers, amino acids, carbohydrates, thioureas, alkaloids, and steroids are some of the categories of compounds that are based on a specific functional group or groups and exhibit almost similar properties. Drugs are classified on the basis of similarity in chemical structure. However, in several cases, the chemical structures of the drugs that have similar therapeutic action are so varied that it is difficult to consider them as being strictly in any one of the functional group categories. Also, drugs with similar chemical structure exhibit different therapeutic properties. In spite of these limitations, this classification is useful to study the chemical properties and synthetic routes of the drugs.

Therapeutic action basis Drugs are classified on the basis of their therapeutic action, into three main classes:

(i) Chemotherapeutic agents
(ii) Pharmacodynamic agents
(iii) Vitamins and Hormones

Chemotherapeutic agents The word chemotherapy may be defined as *the use of drugs in the treatment of infectious diseases, so as to destroy offending parasites or organisms without damaging the host tissues.* Drugs which are used to fight the pathogenic organisms are grouped together as chemotherapeutic agents. A pathogen to be killed inside the human body, is an essential prerequisite for any drug to be classified under this category. Based on the disease the pathogen causes, these drugs are further divided into the following categories (Table 2.1) and the commonly used drugs to combat the disease are provided alongside them.

Table 2.1 *Chemotherapeutic Agents*

Sl. No.	Class of drugs	Disease	Commonly used drugs
1.	Antimalarials	Malaria	chloroquine, quinine
2.	Antibacterials (sulpha drugs)	Bacterial infection	sulphanilamide, sulphadiazine
3.	Antibiotics	Bacterial infection	penicillin G, gentamycin
4.	Antifungals	Fungal	flucanozole, miconazole
5.	Antiprotozoals	Trypanosomiasis	metronidazole, suramin
6.	Antihelmentics	Helminths	niclosamide, quinacrine
7.	Antiseptics	Microorganisms	2-propanol, ethanol, phenol, cresol, resorcinol
8.	Antitubercular drugs	Tuberculosis	isoniazid, rifampin, streptomycin,
9.	Antileprosy drugs	Leprosy	dapsone, thiazolsulfone

Pharmacodynamic agents *Drugs that alter or regulate the biochemistry of the body are said to be pharmacodynamic agents.* Drugs which act selectively on any system of the body like the central nervous system (CNS), peripheral nervous system, cardiovascular system, hematopoietic system, renal system, etc. are refered to as pharmacodynamic agents. These pharamcodynamic agents interact with specific receptors in the body tissues and alter or regulate their biochemical functions. The pharmacodynamic agents are classfied, broadly, into the following types of drugs (Table 2.2) and the site of action of the drug along with the commonly used drugs are indicated below.

There is a detailed discussion about pharmacodynamic agents later on in this chapter.

The relationship between chemical structure and therapeutic actions

The study of the relationship between chemical structure and biological activity involves the synthesis and testing of as many analogs as possible of the *lead drug*. The task of the medicinal chemist is to improve existing drugs by increasing their efficiency and decreasing their side effects, besides creating new drugs through molecular modifications. The study of structure–activity is of great importance in identifying the pharmacophore.

Table 2.2 *Pharmacodynamic Agents*

Sl. No.	Type of drugs	Site of disease	Commonly used drugs
	Drugs acting on the central nervous system (CNS)		
1.	CNS depressants (non-selective)	CNS	morphine, codeine
2.	CNS depressants (selective)	CNS	L-dopa, diazepam, gabapentin
3.	CNS stimulants	CNS	caffeine, LSD, strychnine
4.	Anaesthetics	CNS	thiopental sodium, chloroform, cyclopropane, butacaine
5.	Antipyretics & Analgesics	CNS	aspirin, paracetamol, analgin
	Drugs acting on the peripheral nervous system (PNS)		
6.	Antispasmodics	PNS	atropine, papaverine
7.	Antihistamines	PNS	benadryl, linadryl, antergan
	Drugs acting on the cardiovascular system		
8.	Cardiovascular agents	Heart or blood vessels	digitalis, lidocaine, reserpine
	Drugs acting on the hematopoietic system		
9.	Anticoagulants	Blood	heparin, dicoumarol, 4-hydroxy coumarin, warfarin sodium, aspirin
10	Anti-anemic drugs	Blood	ferrous sulphate, vitamin B_{12}
	Drugs acting on the renal system		
11.	Diuretics	Kidney	bumetanide, chlorothiazide

The physicochemical properties of the drug molecule such as its lipid solubility, partition coefficient, Pka, etc. play an important role in the biological activity. A slight modification in the structure may result in a physiologically more active drug with less side effects. The drug action of a molecule is a function of its chemical constitution.

2.2 *Structure–activity relationship (SAR) in drugs*

Certain features of the chemical structure are related to biological activity. A specific kind of molecular skeleton has a particular type of biological activity (drug property) (Table 2.3). *The biological activity of the drugs is nearly the same for a given type of molecular skeleton, even if there are minor structural and substituent variations and such drugs are called structure-specific drugs.* These drugs have a common type of pharmacophore and can therefore interact with the same receptor.

All sulfanilamides have bacteriostatic activity even when the R-group is varied. Similarly, all arylmethylacetic acids and their derivatives are anti-inflammatory.

Table 2.3 *Molecular Skeleton and Biological Activity*

Sl. No.	Molecular skeleton (pharmacophore)	Class of compounds	Biological activity
1.	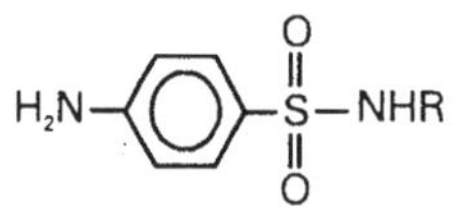	Sulfanilamides	bacteriostatic
2.	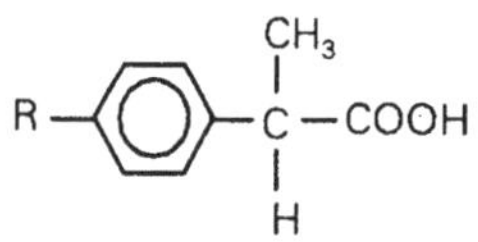	Aryl methylacetic acids	anti-inflammatory
3.	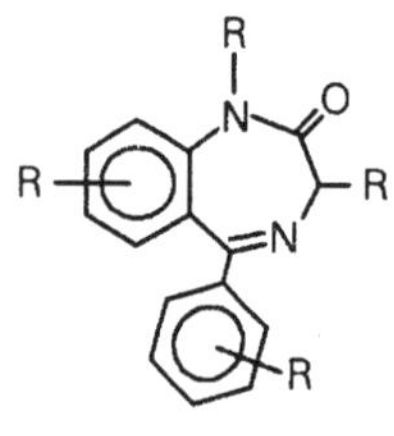	Benzodiazepines	hypnotic and sedative
4.	$Ar_2X-CH_2-CH_2-NR_2$	Dialkylamines	anti-allergic

Lead Structure All drug discovery programmes start with identifying the "lead structure." *A lead drug is the first member of a new class of compounds possessing a good level of drug action for a specific disease.* Prontosil (16) is the lead structure for sulfa antibacterials. Penicillin (52), a β-lactam, is the lead structure for the penicillin class of antibiotics. The lead compound may be identified by synthesizing a large number of compounds and testing them for a specific drug property. It may also be identified by isolating new compounds from plants, bacteria, fungi, etc. and testing them for drug properties. Sometimes, a lead drug is identified serendipitously, e.g., penicillin.

The lead structure itself may be used as a drug, but the medicinal chemist generally tries to improve the activity (potency, site specificity,

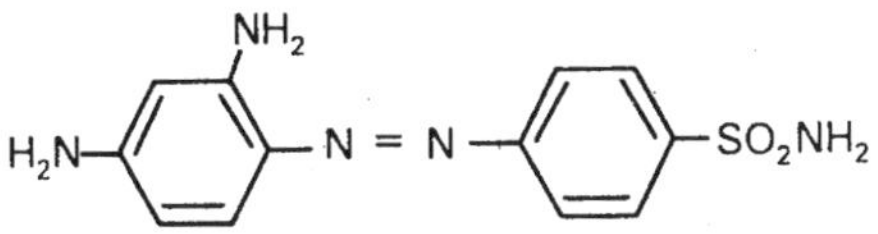

Prontosil (16)

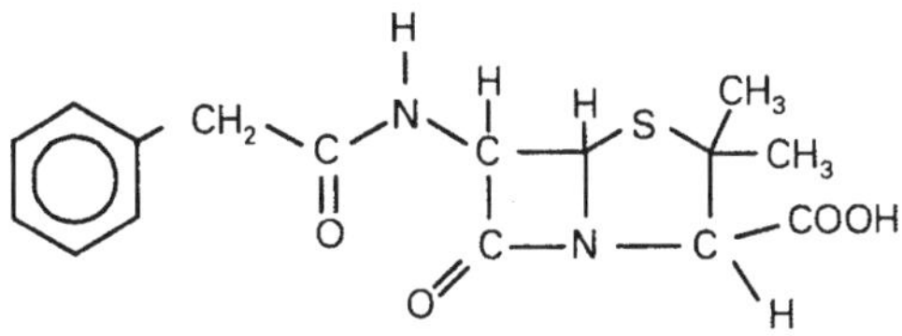

Penicillin (52)

stability, freedom from side effects, etc.) by variation or modification of the lead structure. The modification of the lead structure is generally achieved by: (i) variation of the substituent, (ii) position of the substituent, (iii) change of the ring system, etc. The resulting lead-modified structures are known as *lead analogs*. During these studies, often extending over a period of 5–10 years (after the lead is identified), a very large number (sometimes even 20,000) of lead analogs are synthesized, their drug property evaluated and the relationship between the structures of the lead analogs and their drug property is established. These studies are known as structure–activity relationship (SAR) studies. From such a study, one gets valuable information regarding the (1) ring system, (2) position of the substituent, and (3) electron-releasing or electron-withdrawing nature of the substituent, essential for the maximum drug property. In other words, this study identifies the pharmacophore. Normally, out of the 10,000 or so compounds involved in a SAR study, two or three compounds may be identified and marketed as useful drugs. From penicillin as the lead structure, the drugs ampicillin (19) and amoxicillin (20) were discovered. Similarly, from prontosil as the lead, the sulfa drugs such as sulfadiazine (18), sulfamethoxazole (43), and sulfapyridine were discovered.

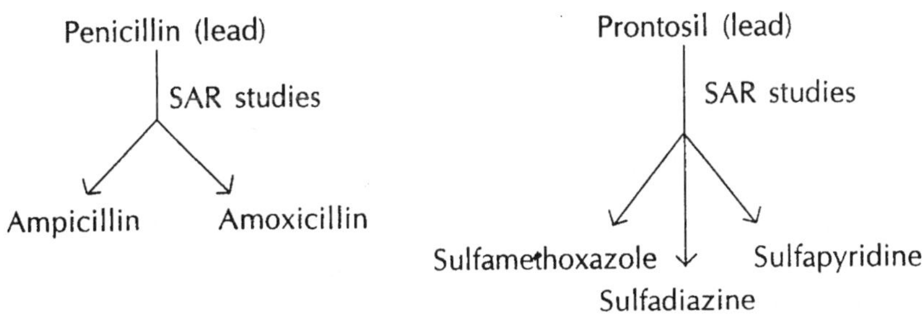

Fig. 2.1 *Drugs discovered from the lead structures.*

Example 1 Structure–activity relationships in antibacterial sulfa drugs

Prontosil is the lead structure. Several thousands of analogs of this compound were synthesized and tested for activity. High bacteriostatic activity was found in the compounds with the general structure (53).

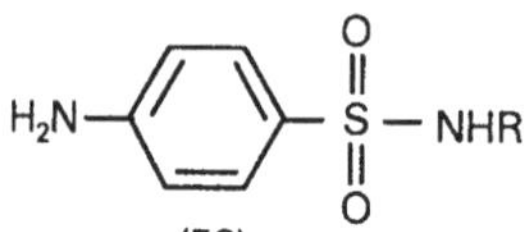

(53)

The following structure to activity relationships were discovered from these studies:

(i) The amine and the sulfonyl groups on the benzene ring should be para. If these substituents are ortho or meta, there is no drug property. With any substituent other than amino group at para position, such as $-CH_3$, $-OH$, $-SO_3H$, $-COOH$, $-Cl$, there is no antibacterial activity.

(ii) The aniline amino group may be unsubstituted or may have a substituent that is removed *in vivo*.

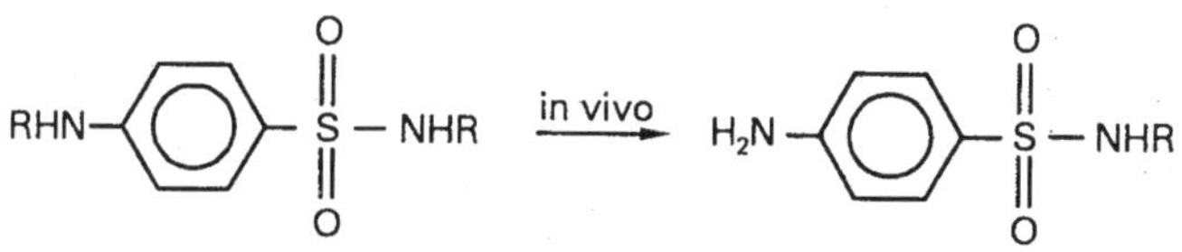

If the substituent on the aniline amino group cannot be converted to free $-NH_2$ *in vivo*, there is no drug activity.

(iii) The replacement of the benzene ring by other ring systems or the introduction of an additional substituent on it, decreases the potency or abolishes the activity.

(iv) 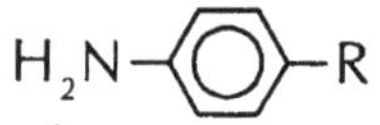 The R group may be $-SO_2$ 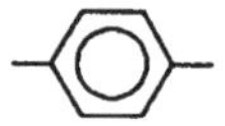 NH_2, 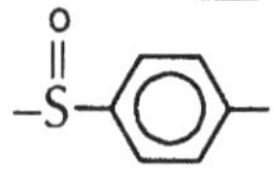 NH_2, $-C(=O)-NH_2$, $-CONHR$, 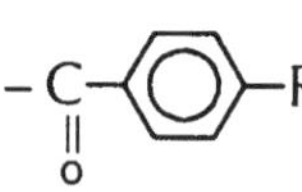 R, but the potency is reduced in most cases.

(v) 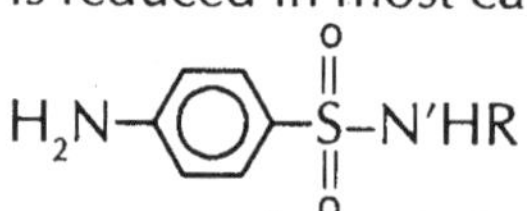 N′ mono-substitution results in more potent compounds and the potency increases with a heteroaromatic substituent (oxazole, pyridine, diazine, etc.).

(vi) 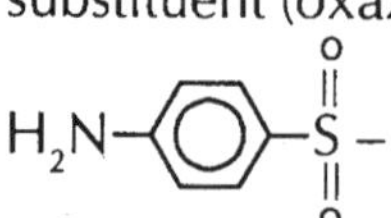 : N′ disubstitution generally leads to inactive compounds.

The above statements 1 to 6 are the result of SAR studies of the sulfa drug analogs. From the 10,000 or so compounds synthesized, (i) Sulfadiazine (18), (ii) Sulfamethoxazole (43), and (iii) Sulfapyridine have been discovered.

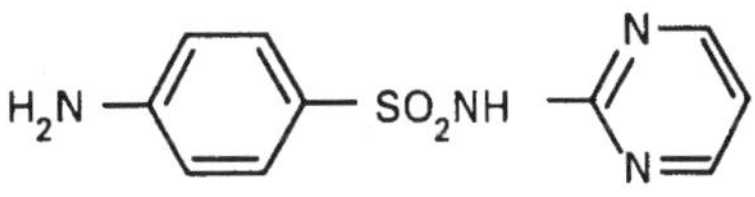

Sulfadiazine (18)

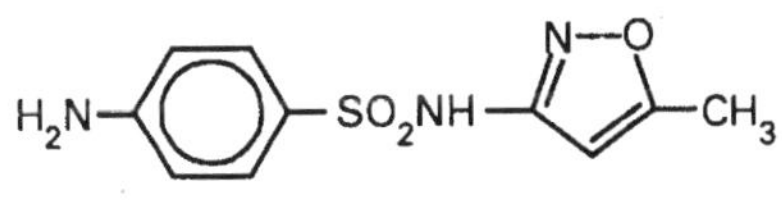

Sulfamethoxazole (43)

Example 2 Structure-activity studies in sleep-inducing (hypnotics-sedatives) benzodiazepenes.

The lead structure, Librium (34), was discovered serendipitiously by Dr. Leo Sternbach of La Roche laboratories. About 2000 compounds, analogs of librium (54), were synthesized and tested and the following structure–activity relationships were discovered.

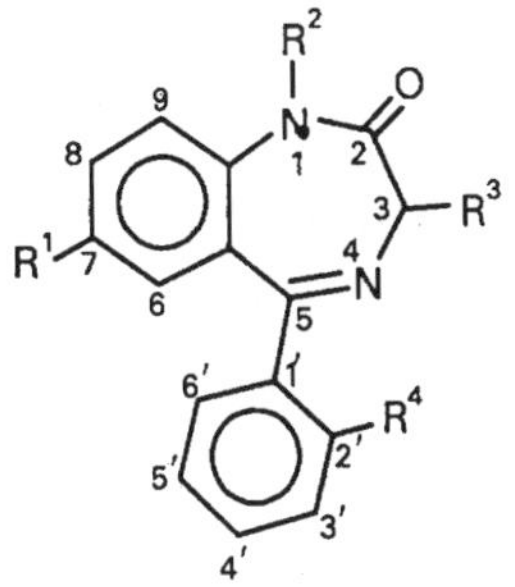

(54)

(i) Electron-withdrawing substituents (Cl, Br, NO_2, CF_3, CN, etc) at 7 position (R^1) confer high activity. Larger groups or electron donor substituents decrease activity.

(ii) Any substituent (electron releasing or withdrawing, small or large) at C–6, C–8, C–9 positions decrease potency.

(iii) 3-Hydroxy compounds show comparable potency, whereas 3-alkyl groups reduce potency (R^3).

(iv) Hydrogenation of the double bond at 4–5 position reduces the activity.

(v) A phenyl group at C–5 position is necessary for activity. Only halogens Cl, F, Br at C–2′ position enhance potency, and other substituents at C–3′, 4′, 5′ decrease activity.

(vi) The replacement of C–2 lactam oxygen by sulphur decreases activity.

(vii) Alkyl substitution at N^1 is not necessary.

From the 2000 analogs of librium synthesized and tested, the following valuable hypnotic-sedative drugs, diazepam (12), lorazepam (55) and chlorazepam (56), have been discovered.

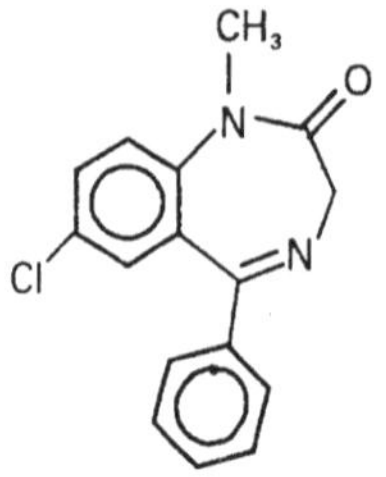

Diazepam (12)

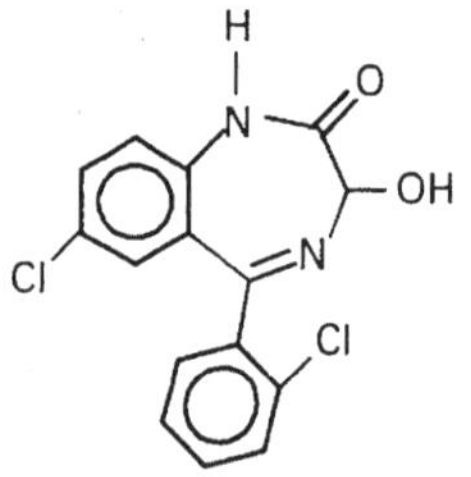

Lorazepam (55)

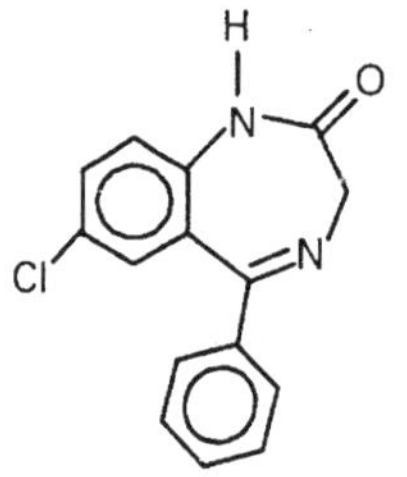

Chlorazepam (56)

Pharmacodynamic agents

2.3 Drugs acting on the central nervous system (CNS)

The nervous system in the body is responsible for the transmission of information. The major anatomical parts of the CNS are the brain, cerebellum, medulla and spinal cord. Functionally, all the parts of the CNS which are concerned with one type of activity are interlinked. It is now known that several endogenous chemicals play a transmitter role in the functioning of the CNS. The fundamental unit of the CNS is the neuron or nerve cell. The human body contains several billion neurons. Each neuron exhibits varied and highly complex activity. Broadly, the various functions that are attended to by the CNS include memory; fine voluntary movements; judgement; discrimination; special senses like vision, smell and hearing; thinking; integration of emotional behaviour; coordination and control of body posture; perception of pain; temperature and touch (senses); control of the autonomic nervous system; behaviour (sexual, eating, drinking, sleeping, etc.); respiration; swallowing, vomiting, and reflex movements. Any malfunctioning of the neurons may lead to a disease. Therefore, drugs can play a significant role in the maintenance and in setting right the disorders of the CNS. Drugs acting on the CNS are also termed as **psychopharmacological agents**.

Classification The drugs which affect the CNS may be divided into three broad categories. They are:

(i)Non-selective CNS depressants, (ii) Non-selective CNS stimulants, and (iii) Selective modifiers of CNS.

i. **Non-selective CNS Depressants** Depressants are drugs which reduce the activity of the CNS. These drugs depress the nervous system and exert their effect in a non-selective way. This category includes general anaesthetics, sedatives and hypnotics, antipyretics, analgesics, and antirheumatics.

ii. **Non-selective CNS stimulants** Stimulants are drugs which activate the CNS. These drugs exert their action non-selectively by direct neuronal excitation. Analeptics, anxiolytics, antidepressants and psychotomimetics (hallucinogens) are the major categories that come under this group.

iii. **Selective modifiers of CNS** The drugs in this category may manifest either depressant or stimulant effects. The principal classes of drugs under selective modifiers include anticonvulsants (antiepileptics), antitussives, antiparkinsonian drugs and neuroleptics.

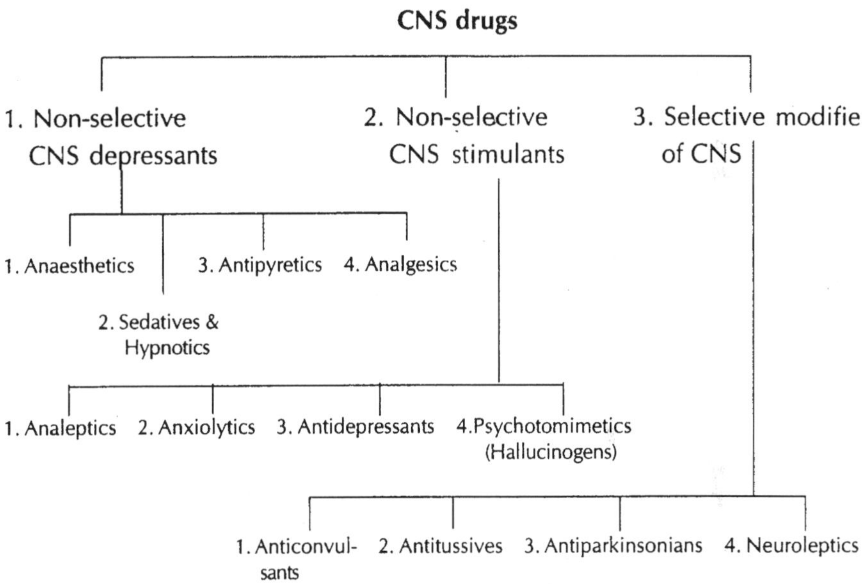

Fig. 2.2 *Classification of CNS drugs.*

2.3.1 Non-selective CNS depressants

2.3.1.1 Anaesthetics

An anaesthetic is defined *as a drug that causes a temporary loss of sensation with or without loss of consciousness*. A wide range of drugs with diverse chemical structures act as anesthetics. Historically, Horace Wells (Hartford), a dentist, introduced nitrous oxide as an anaesthetic in surgery in the year 1844, which was followed by use of ether by William Morton (Boston), and the use of chloroform by James Simpson (Edinburgh). In general, an ideal anaesthetic should have the following characteristics. It should be: (i) non-inflammable, (ii) inexpensive, (iii) require uncomplicated equipment for administration, (iv) provide sufficient muscular relaxation, (v) have no effect on the myocardium or respiration at anaesthetic doses, (vi) chemically and metabolically stable, (vii) sufficiently potent to permit adequate oxygen supply, and (viii) have a wide margin of safety. Anaesthetics are broadly divided into two groups: (i) General Anaesthetics, and (ii) Local Anaesthetics (Fig. 2.3).

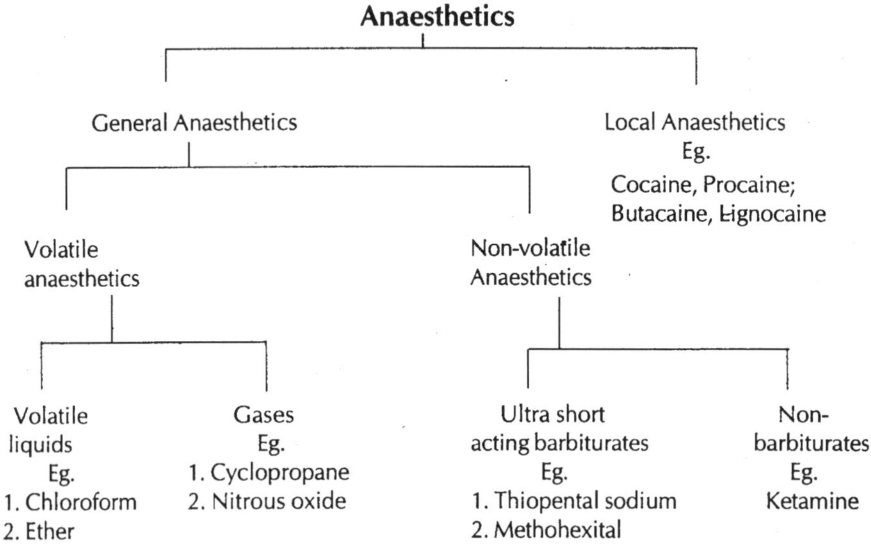

Fig. 2.3 *Classification of anaesthatics.*

Besides these general and local anaesthetics, many CNS depressants, such as analgesics and muscle relaxants, also come under this category.

General Anaesthetics These are CNS depressant drugs that produce partial or total loss of the sensation of pain, which may be accompanied by a loss of consciousness. This state of insensibility is known as anesthesia. Before the advent of effective anaesthetic agents, individuals were prepared for surgery by several subhuman methods such as tying the patient with ropes, giving large doses of alcohol or opium, etc. Painless surgery became a reality only after the chemists prepared synthetic anaesthetics.

For a long time, ethyl ether, chloroform and nitrous oxide (N_2O) were used as anaesthetics. Ether is inflammable and when it combines with air, oxygen, or nitrous oxide, it becomes explosive. When ether is used, the recovery is prolonged and is often accompanied by nausea and vomiting. Ether irritates the respiratory tract, resulting in excessive salivation and secretion of bronchial mucus. The use of chloroform as an anaesthetic is severely restricted because of its narrow margin of safety and its toxicity to the liver and kidneys. Nitrous oxide (N_2O), popularly known as laughing gas, has been discarded now due to its side effects, such as myocardial contractility due to its direct action on the heart.

More recently, fluorinated ethers or hydrocarbons have been introduced (Table 2.4), which have overcome most of the problems associated with classical volatile anaesthetics like ether and chloroform. The presence of fluorine atoms decreases inflammability.

Table 2.4 *Fluorinated Anaesthetics*

Generic Name	Trade Name	Structural formula
Desflurane	Suprane	$CHF_2 - O - CHF - CF_3$
Enflurane	Ethrane	$CHF_2 - O - CF_2 - CHFCl$
Halothane	Fluothane	$CF_3 - CHBrCl$
Isoflurane	Forane	$CHF_2 - O - CHCl - CF_3$
Sevoflurane	—	$(CF_3)_2\, CH - O - CH_2F$

Local Anaesthetics The anaesthesia produced by local anaesthetics is generally without loss of consciousness or the impairment of vital central functions. For this reason, local anaesthetics play an important role clinically in dentistry and in other minor surgeries for temporary relief from pain. *Local anaesthetics are drugs that cause a state of loss of sensation by reversibly blocking the nerve impulses that transmit the feeling of pain*

Table 2.5 *Recently Developed Local Anaesthetics*

Generic Name	Proprietory Name Trade Name	Recommended Application
Lidocaine	Xylocaine, Dalcaine, Nervocaine	Parenteral & Topical
Benzocaine	Americaine	Topical
Butacaine (57)	Butyn	Topical
Butamben (58)	Butesin	Topical
Procaine (59)	Novocain	Parenteral

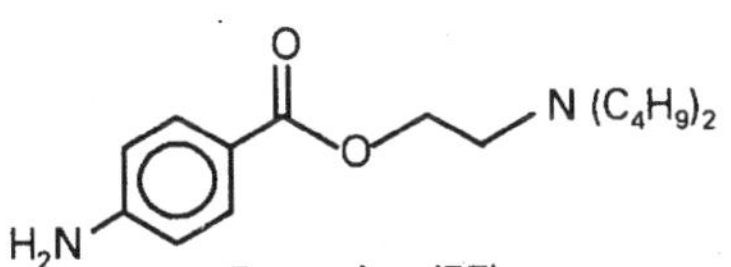

Butacaine (57)

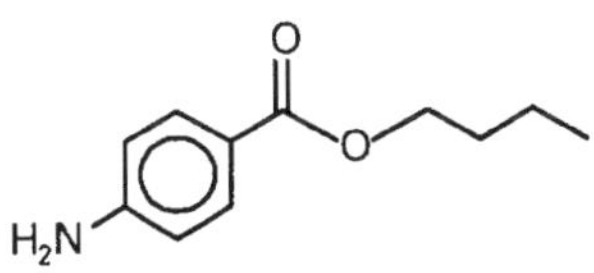

Butamben (58)

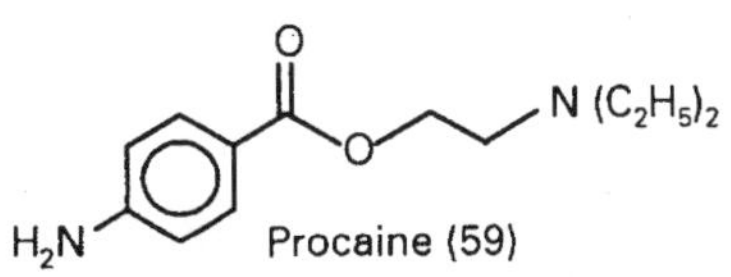

Procaine (59)

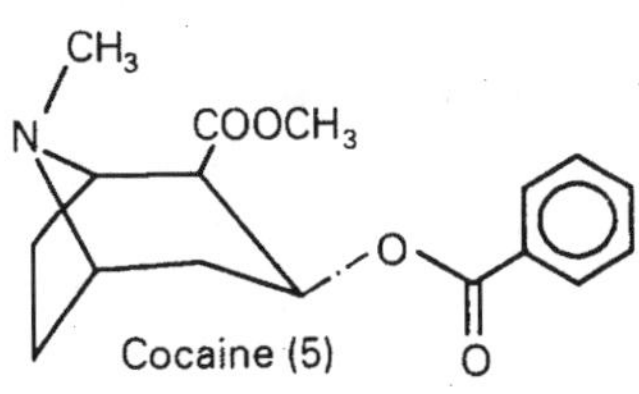

Cocaine (5)

from the particular local area to the brain. Cocaine (5) was the first local anaesthetic that was used as far back as 1880. Unfortunately, cocaine produces side effects like allergic reactions, tissue irritation, and has drawbacks like poor stability in aqueous solution and easy decomposibility.

The clinically available local anaesthetics are given (Table 2.5) along with the recommended mode of application.

2.3.1.2 Sedatives and hypnotics

Sedatives and hypnotics are non-selective CNS depressants. A sedative is used to induce mild relaxation. *A sedative produces mild depression and calms anxiety and excitation, without causing drowsiness or impaired performance. A hypnotic compels the user to sleep, and induces a stronger form of depression.* An anaesthetic produces very strong depression (surgical anesthesia). Drugs can be used for a depressing effect on the CNS in varying degrees, from mild sedation to anaesthesia, depending upon the dose and route of administration.

Sedation brings about a state of depression or calmness. It is characterized by consciousness without any loss of the basic reflexes. Sedation is a rapidly reversible state and sensory stimulation quickly brings about a full arousal of senses. On the other hand, hypnosis (use of a hypnotic drug) is characterized by a temporary loss of arousability and reflex action. This depression is deeper than that of sedation. The sedative and hypnotic drugs are a wide variety of chemical compounds, which include barbiturates (butabarbital, phenobarbital) (7), benzodiazepines (diazepam (12), lorazepam (55), chlorazepam (56)), acetylene derivatives (ethchlorvynol) and aldehydes (chloral hydrate, and paraldehyde). It is to be noted that some of these drugs, when administered in small doses, cause sedation, larger doses cause hypnosis, and still larger doses bring about surgical anaesthesia.

Patient $\rightleftharpoons$ Sedation $\rightleftharpoons$ Hypnosis $\rightleftharpoons$ Anaesthesia $\rightleftharpoons$ Coma $\longrightarrow$ Death

For many centuries, the only sleep-inducing drugs known were alcohol and opium. Today, many compounds capable of producing sleep are available. The first hypnotic barbiturate, barbital (63), was introduced by Fischer in 1903 under the trade name of veronal. The second oldest barbiturate is phenobarbital (7). Barbituric acid (62) is synthesized from urea and malonic acid (Fig. 2.4) and is not itself a CNS depressant. The derivatives of barbituric acid obtained by replacing the two hydrogens on the carbon atom, in position 5 by alkyl or aryl groups, are called barbiturates and have hypnotic property.

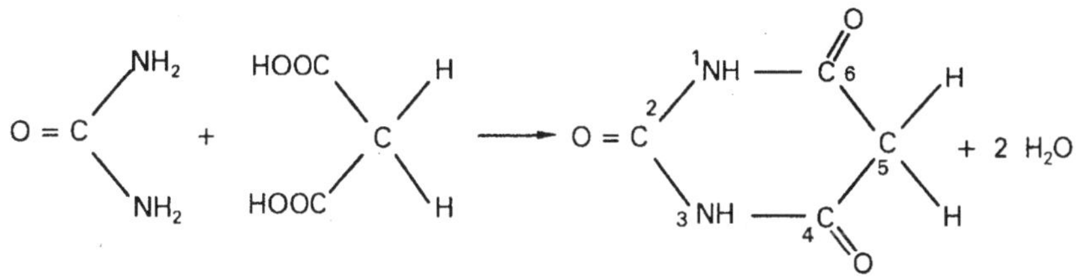

Urea (60) Malonic acid (61) Barbituric acid (62)

Fig. 2.4 *Synthesis of barbituric acid.*

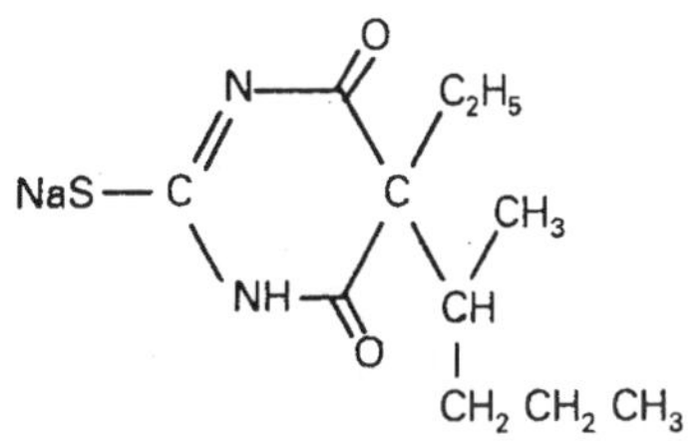

Thiopental Sodium (6)
(Pentothal Sodium)

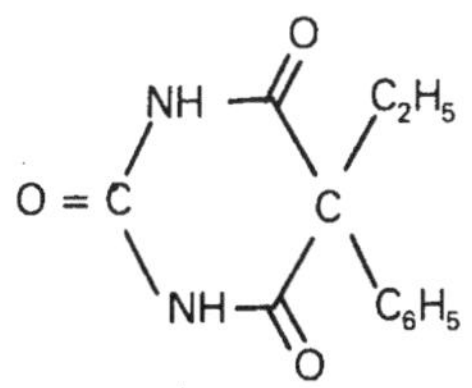

Phenobarbital (7)
(Luminal)

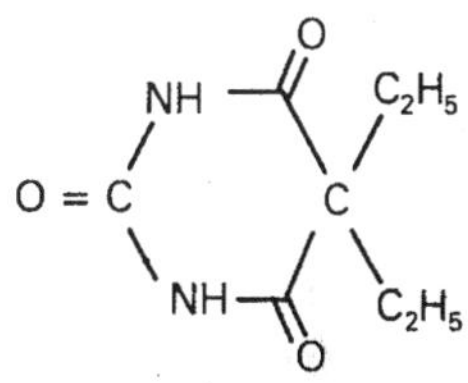

Barbital (63)
(Veronal)

Benzodiazepines act as hypnotics and a major advantage is their relative safety. The tendency of benzodiazepines to interact with other drugs is smaller than that of barbiturates. The disadvantages of benzodiazepine appears to be the slowness of its elimination, and its addictive quality.

Acetylene derivatives, like ethchlorvynol (64), are mild hypnotic drugs with a quick onset and short duration activity. Ethchlorvynol also has anticonvulsant and muscle relaxing properties. It may induce habit and tolerance. The sedative dose is 100 to 200 mg; the hypnotic dose is 500 mg.

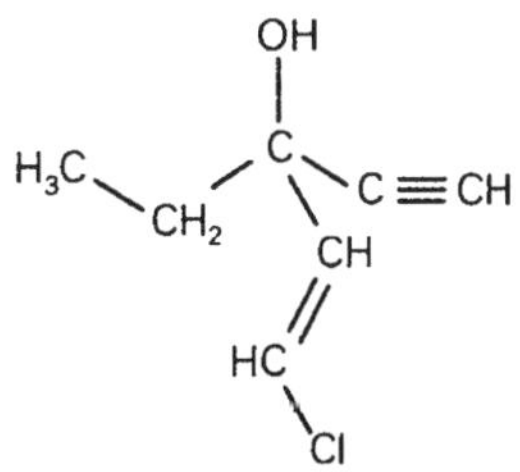

Ethchlorvynol (64)

Liebreich introduced chloral hydrate (65) (a crystalline, water-soluble hydrate), and this was followed by paraldehyde (66) (a trimer of acetaldehyde). Chloral hydrate is a common adulterant in country liquor.

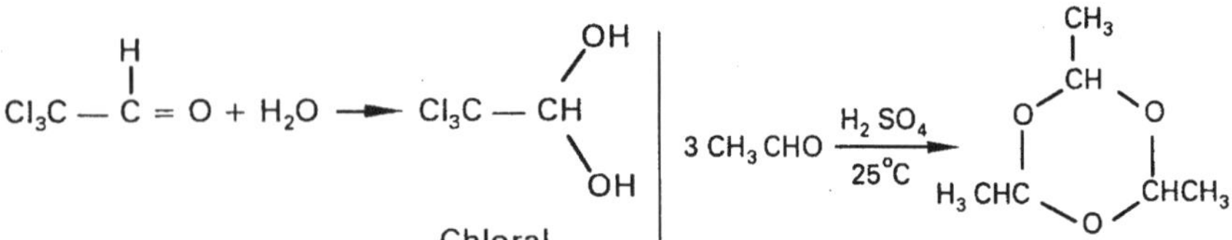

Chloral hydrate (65)

Paraldehyde (66)

Fig. 2.5 *Synthesis of chloral hydrate and paraldehyde.*

2.3.1.3 Antipyretics

An antipyretic is a drug that restores normal body temperature in the presence of fever. The CNS, particularly the hypothalamus (part of the brain above the pituitary gland) which functions like a 'thermostat', maintains the balance between heat production and heat loss to regulate body temperature. The average normal oral body temperature is about 98.4°F or 36.7°C. Antipyretic drugs, when administered to a patient suffering with fever, activate the hypothalamic centers, dilate the peripheral blood vessels, and increase the rate of perspiration. This causes the body to lose heat and thereby lowers the temperature. In most instances, antipyretic therapy by itself is not needed except for reasons of comfort. Antipyretics have no effect on the normal body temperature and also do not affect the infectious causes of fever. Antipyretic agents also have mild analgesic activity. The antipyretic—analgesic drugs may be divided into three classes.

(i) **Salicylates**

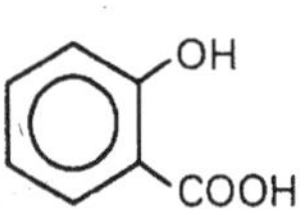

Salicylic acid (67)

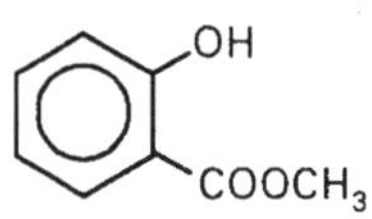

Methyl salicylate (68)

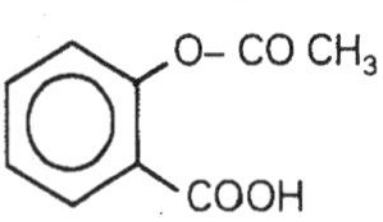

Aspirin (1)

(ii) **Para-aminophenol derivatives**

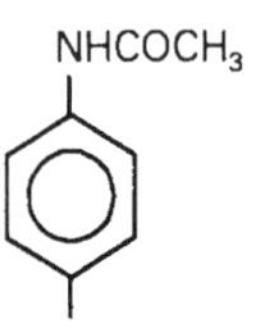

Phenacetin (69)

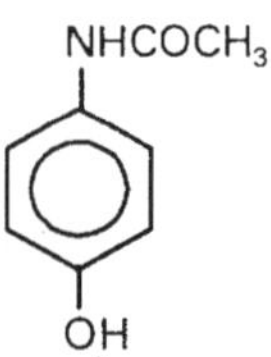

Acetaminophen (9)
(paracetamol)

(iii) **Pyrazolone derivatives**

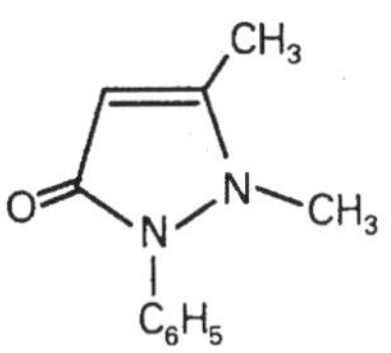

Antipyrine (70)

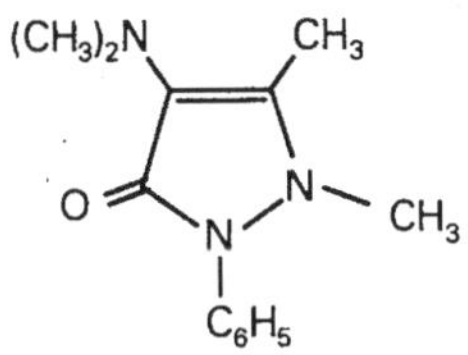

Aminopyrine (71)

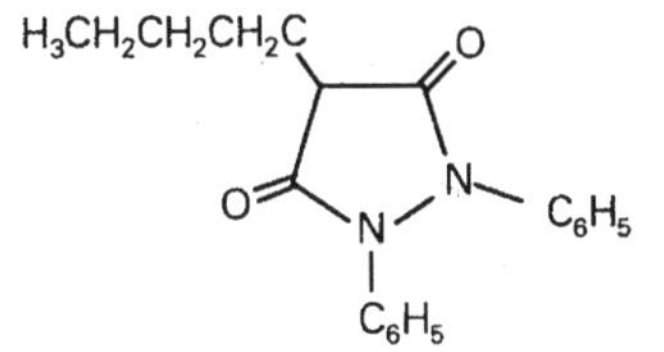

Phenylbutazone (8)

Aspirin (1) or paracetamol (acetaminophen) (9) is quite effective in reducing fever. The synthesis and other therapeutic details of some of these compounds are given in Chapter 3.

2.3.1.4 Analgesics

Drugs that relieve pain without significantly imparing consciousness are called analgesics. Analgesics are also known as analgetics. They act on the CNS and decrease the sensation of pain. Most commonly, pain can be due to headache, neuralgia, chronic arthritis, labour, stomachache, or cardiac, muscular, traumatic and pressure reasons. The main action of analgesics is to decrease the sensation of pain and act by increasing the threshold of pain. *The threshold of pain is defined as the lowest perceptible intensity of pain.* The pain is induced by a stimulus in a cell, tissue or other structures of the body. The amount of stimulus may be regarded as a measure of the threshold of pain. If greater stimulus is required to produce the pain, the threshold of pain is said to be higher and if less stimulus is needed, the pain threshold is said to be low. When analgesics are used, the pain is not decreased but the threshold of pain is increased. Therefore, the patient does not feel the pain or is able to tolerate the pain.

Analgesics are grouped into two classes: (i) non-narcotic agents, and (ii) narcotic agents.

Non-narcotic analgesics The non-narcotic analgesics are antipyretic and anti-inflammatory painkillers. All antipyretic drugs are also used as analgesics. Aspirin, paracetamol, analgin and ibuprofen are some of the commonly used, good, non-narcotic analgesics. These drugs act centrally or sometimes peripherally, by blocking impulse generation at the receptors mediating pain.

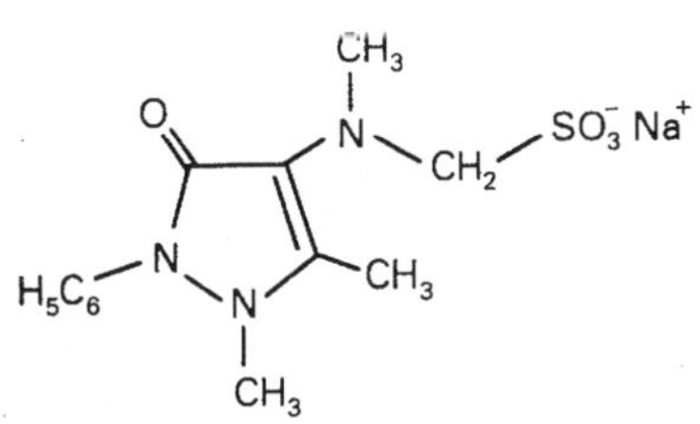

Analgin (10)

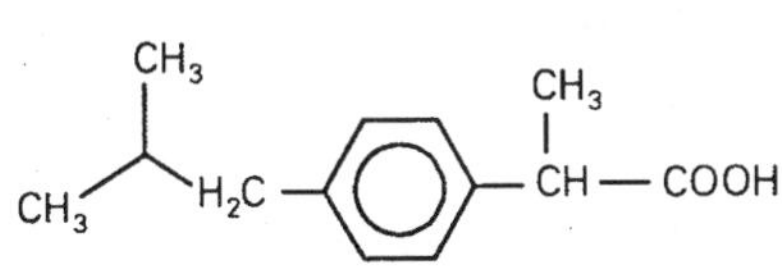

Ibuprofen (11)

NSAIDs Inflammation usually means pain with a burning sensation, in any part of the body or tissues. Non-Steroidal Anti-Inflammatory Drugs (NSAIDs) possess anti-inflammatory properties in addition to antipyretic and analgesic properties, which are useful in the treatment of certain rheumatic disorders (note: all analgesic-antipyretic drugs may not have anti-inflammatory activity). Since these drugs possess a non-steroidal structure and yet relieve pain, they are termed NSAIDs. These NSAIDs are very effective in the control of moderate pain of various musculo-skeletal disorders, menstrual cramps, and moderate post-operative discomfort. These drugs act by inhibiting the biosynthesis of prostaglandins. Aspirin (1), acetaminophen (paracetamol) (9), ibuprofen (11), naproxen (47), ketoprofen (48), sulindac (37) and nabumetone (72), and diclofenac (73) are some of the most commonly used NSAIDs.

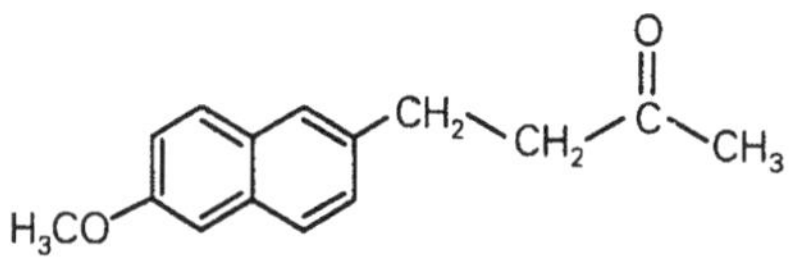

Nabumetone (Relafen) (72)

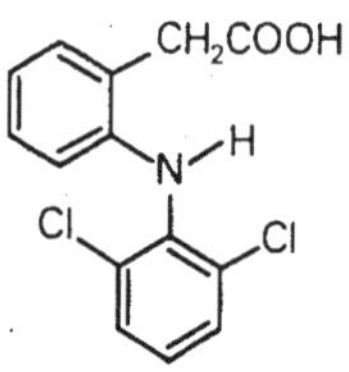

Diclofenac (73)

Narcotic analgesics Historically, opioid analgesics have been called 'narcotic analgesics'. Narcotic analgesic literally means that these agents cause sleep or loss of consciousness, in addition to their pain-relieving effect. The juice (opium in Greek) or gum from the unripe seed-pods of the poppy, *Papaver somniferum,* is among the oldest medications recorded. The pharmacist, Surturnev, first isolated an alkaloid from opium in the year 1803. He named the 'alkaloid' morphine (74), after Morpheus, the Greek God of dreams. Codeine (75), thebaine (76), and papaverine (77) are other medically important alkaloids that were later isolated from opium gum.

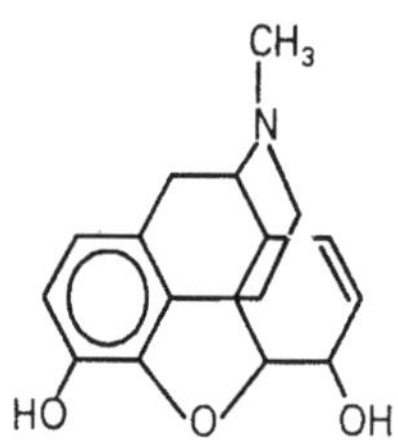

Morphine (74)

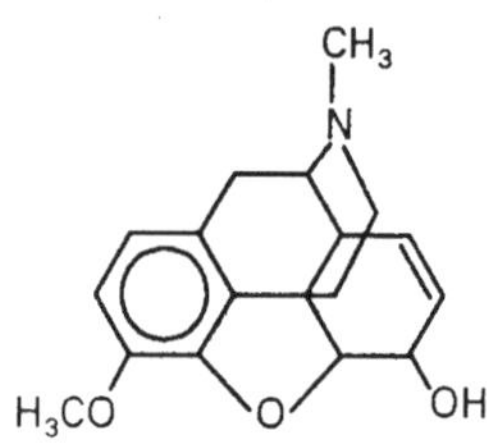

Codeine (75)

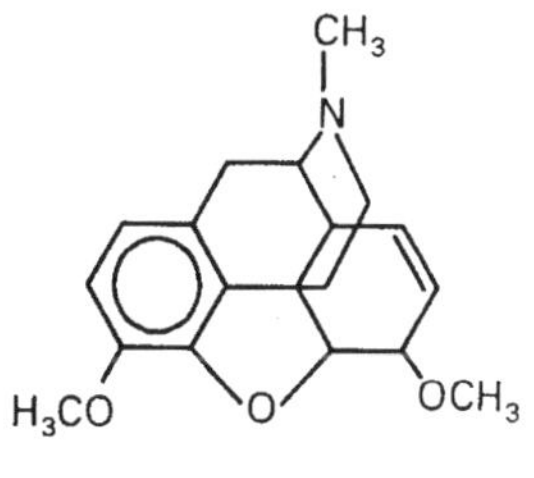

Thebaine (76)

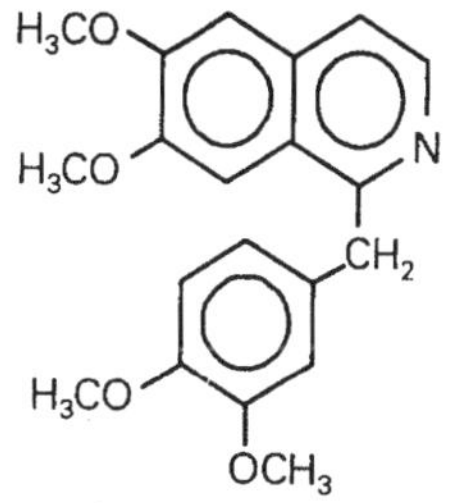

Papaverine (77)

Opioid analgesics are used for moderate to severe pain that cannot be relieved with other agents. Increasing tolerance and dependancy are normal consequences of opioid therapy. This should not be confused with addiction. While addiction is a psychological dependency, generally referred to as 'drug abuse', the opioid drugs may be a physiological necessity. *Drug abuse is defined as manipulative drug-seeking behaviour or the compulsive use of drugs for non-medicinal purposes, despite harmful side-effects.* Patients with chronic, severe pain must not consider themselves addicts just because they are being treated with opioids. (Patients and their family members must be educated regarding the difference between tolerance, physical dependence and addiction).

The World Health Organisation (WHO) recommends a 3-step method for the use of analgesics. In step-1, the agents used for mild to moderate pain, are non-opioids such as aspirin, acetaminophen or NSAIDs. If pain persists or increases, step-2 adds an opioid to the non-opioid. If pain still continues or intensifies, step-3 increases the opioid potency or dosage, while continuing the non-opioid.

2.3.2 Non-selective CNS stimulants

CNS Stimulants (Psychoactive Drugs) Some people suffer from emotional problems like anxiety, tension, fear, loneliness, etc., leading to neuroses. *The drugs which primarily affect mental processes to improve moods are called psychoactive drugs* and, hence, are classified under CNS stimulants. If given in high doses, they may cause psychosis. Neurosis and psychosis are mental illnesses which are associated with psychological disorders involving the brain. The difference is that in the case of neurosis the insight (ability of a patient to realize that he is ill) is retained, whereas in psychosis one loses contact with reality. A prolonged CNS stimulation always results in depression. The CNS stimulants can be categorized into 4 groups depending on their clinical use (Fig. 2.6). They are: (i) Analeptics, (ii) Anxiolytics, (iii) Antidepressants, and (iv) Psychotomimetics.

General CNS stimulants

Analeptics Eg.	Anxiolytics Eg.	Antidepressants Eg.	Psychotomimetics (Hallucinogens) Eg.
1) Caffeine	1) Librium	1) Imipramine	1) LSD
2) Strychnine	2) Valium	2) Amitriptyline	2) Mescaline
3) Nikethamide	3) Prazepam (Verstran)	3) Opipramol	3) Amphetamine
4) Amphetamine		4) Iproniazid	4) Psilocybin
5) Ethamivan		5) Phenelzine	

Fig. 2.6 *Classification of general CNS stimulants.*

2.3.2.1 Analeptics

Analeptics are a class of CNS stimulants which excite the medullary centres when they are in a depressed state and improve the metabolic activity of the brain. Analeptics are used for certain respiratory diseases, post-anesthetic respiratory problems, circulatory failure causing low blood pressure, and to counter an overdose of barbiturates, narcotics, analgesics, and general anaesthetics. Caffeine (78), a xanthine derivative, stimulates the cardiac muscles, enhances diuresis, bronchi and coronary arteries. The other drugs include, nikethamide (coramine) (79), ethamivan, (emivan) (80) and amphetamine (benzedrine) (81).

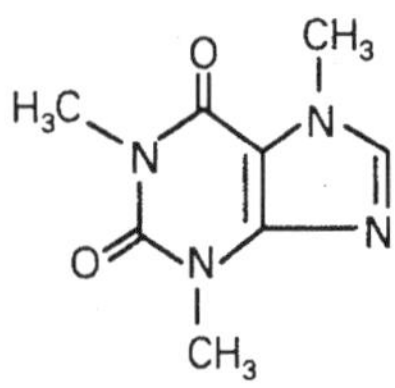

Caffeine (78)

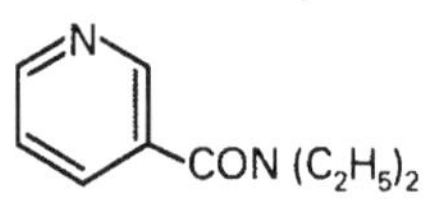

Nikethamide (79)
(Coramine)

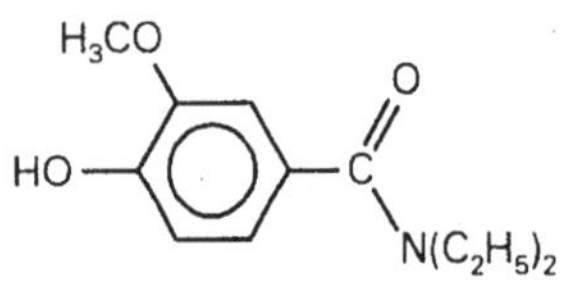

Ethamivan (80)
(Emivan)

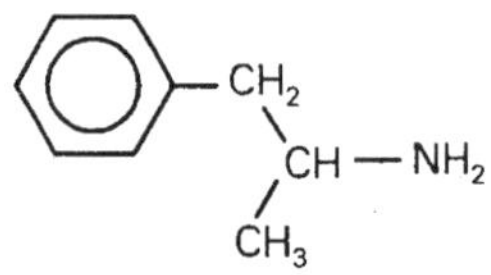

Amphetamine (81)
(Benzedrine)

2.3.2.2 Anxiolytics

Anxiolytics include tranquillizers, relaxants and antineurotic agents, and are mood stabilizers which act on the brain. They include: (i) chlordiazepoxide (librium) (34), (ii) diazepam (valium) (12), and (iii) prazepam (verstran; centrax).

2.3.2.3 Antidepressants

Antidepressants are drugs that are used on patients who suffer from acute mental depression. These drugs are CNS stimulants as they elevate the mood and generally have no effect on normal persons. They do have side effects such as dryness of the mouth, blurred vision, constipation and urinary problems. Because of their sedative effect, they are usually used at bedtime. Antidepressants include (i) imipramine (82), (ii) amitriptyline (83), (iii) nortriptyline (84) and (iv) fluoxetine (prozac) (85). Nortriptyline, which is a metabolic product of amytriptyline, is twice as potent as an antidepressant. Fluoxetine (prozac) (85) is also known as the "Happiness pill". The chief advantage of fluoxetine is that it does not cause significant cardiovascular side effects or weight-gain.

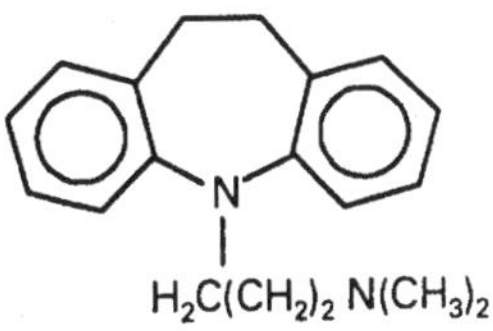

Imipramine (82)
(Tofranil)

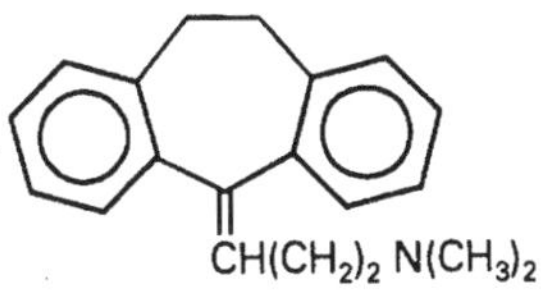

Amitriptyline (83)
(Elavil)

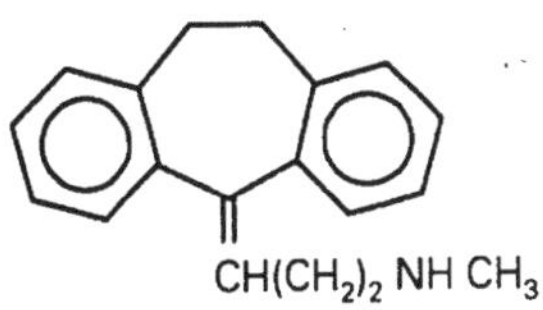

Nortriptyline (84)
(Aventil)

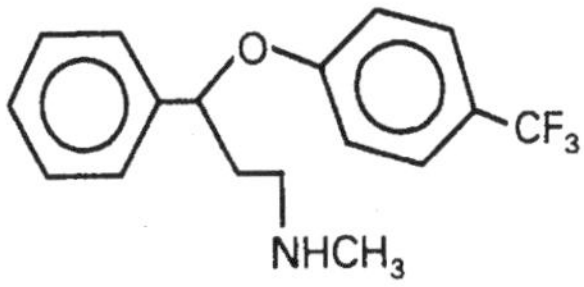

Fluoxetine (85)
(Prozac)

2.3.2.4 Psychotomimetics (Hallucinogens)

Psychotomimetic drugs are used for mental illness. The effects of these drugs include disturbed perception, hallucinations, the feeling of weightlessness, vision of patterns of colour and loss of memory. These drugs are habit-forming if used repeatedly. They include LSD (lysergic acid diethylamide) (delysid) (86), mescaline (peyote). These drugs should only be used under a doctor's supervision.

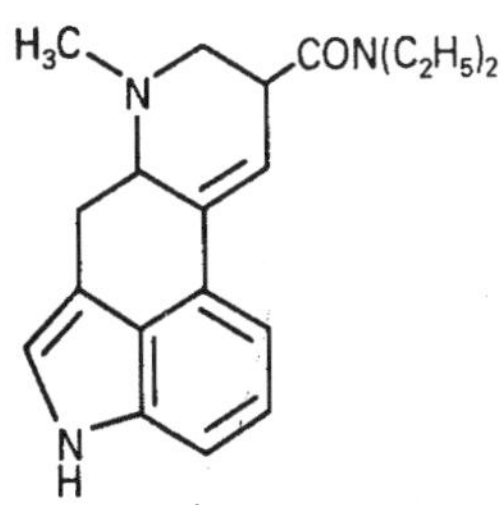

LSD (86)
(Delysid)

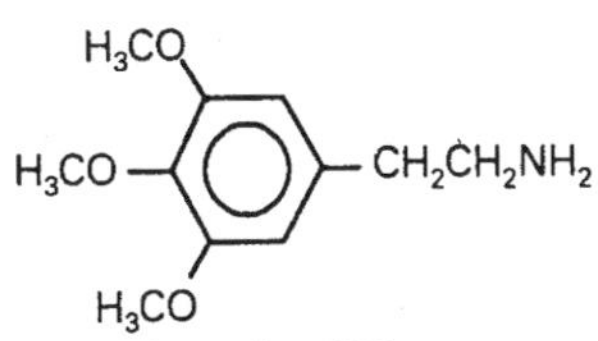

Mescaline (87)
(Peyote)

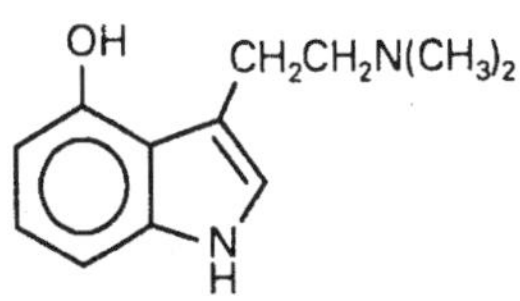

Psilocybin (88)

2.3.3 Selective modifiers of CNS

The drugs related to selective modifiers of CNS include both depressants and stimulants and are categorized into four groups (Fig. 2.7). The commonly used drugs are also indicated.

Selective modifiers of CNS

Anticonvulsants or anti-epileptics	Antitussives	Antiparkinsonians	Neuroleptics
Eg.	Eg.	Eg.	Eg.
1) Gabapentin	1) Noscapine	1) Levodopa	1) Chlorpromazine
2) Diazepam	2) Pholcodine	2) Carbidopa	2) Haloperidol
3) Primidone	3) Dextromethorphan		3) Loxapine
4) Phenytoin			4) Molindone
5) Valproic acid			

Fig. 2.7 *Classification of selective modifiers of CNS.*

2.3.3.1 Anticonvulsants

In the middle ages, epilepsy (convulsions or fits) was considered to be due to the presence of an evil spirit in the affected individual, and the treatment was also according to this belief. The term 'epilepsy' is based on the Greek word 'epilambanein' (meaning 'to seize'), and was first mentioned by Hippocrates. *Epilepsy is broadly defined as a CNS disease characterized by recurring seizure disorders (fits).* It is manifested as a sudden loss or disturbance of consciousness (but not always), and characteristic body movements (convulsions). It is characterized as primary or idiopathic when there is no known cause for the seizure, and secondary or symptomatic when the cause or origin of the disease (etiology) has been identified. Symptomatic epilepsy can result from specific physiological phenomena such as brain tumours, syphillis, cerebral

Table 2.6 *Common Drugs for Epilepsy*

Year introduced	Generic or Non-proprietory name	Trade name
1912	Phenobarbital (7)	Luminal
1951	Phenacemide (89)	Phenurone
1954	Primidone (90)	Mysoline
1968	Diazepam (12)	Valium
1994	Gabapentin (91)	Neurontin
—	Phenytoin (92)	Dilantin
—	Valproic Acid (93)	—

arteriosclerosis, multiple sclerosis (nervous disease), sunstroke, acute intoxication, lead poisoning, vitamin B_6 deficiency, hypoglycemia and labour. All forms of epilepsy originate in the brain and is believed to be the result of changes in neuronal activity. Some of the anti-epileptic drugs that are in common use are given in Table 2.6. Many anticonvulsant drugs are non-specific depressants of the CNS.

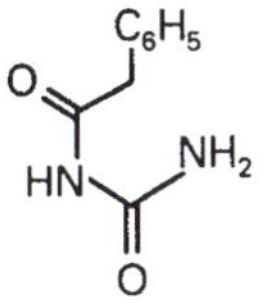

Phenacemide
(89)

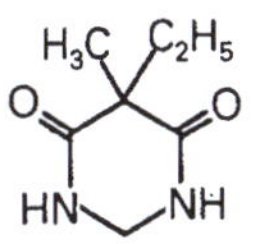

Primidone
(90)

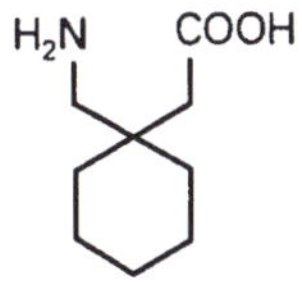

Gabapentin
(91)

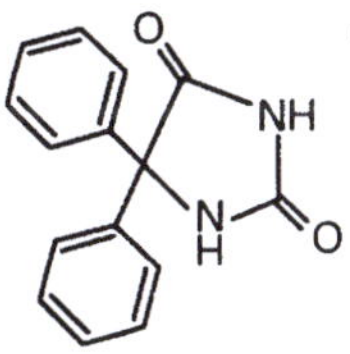

Phenytoin
(92)

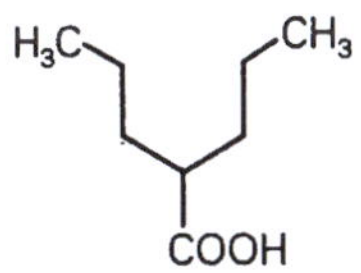

Valproic Acid
(93)

2.3.3.2 Antitussives

Drugs which are used to suppress irritating coughs are called antitussives. A cough is a physiological mechanism, used to clear the respiratory tract from foreign material. It should not be suppressed indiscriminately. However, there are situations where a cough irritates the patient or leads to insomnia. In such situations, one may use a drug that will reduce the frequency or intensity of the coughing. There are two types of antitussives: (i) centrally acting, and (ii) peripherally acting.

Centrally-acting antitussives include opium alkaloids. Many of the narcotic analgesics, like codeine (75) and ethyl morphine, are also useful antitussives. Peripheral antitussives comprise of demulcents, expectorants, and mucolytic agents.

Demulcent A soothing agent that protects the mucus membranes and relieves irritation.

Expectorant A drug that enhances the secretion of sputum so that it is easier to cough up and clear the throat.

Mucolytic An agent that breaks down or dissolves excessive or thickened mucus secretions.

Some of the antitussive compounds include noscapine (94), pholcodine (95), and dextromethorphan (96).

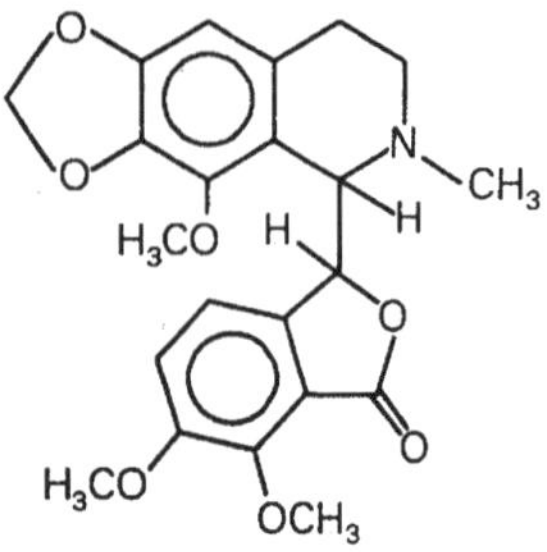

Noscapine (94)

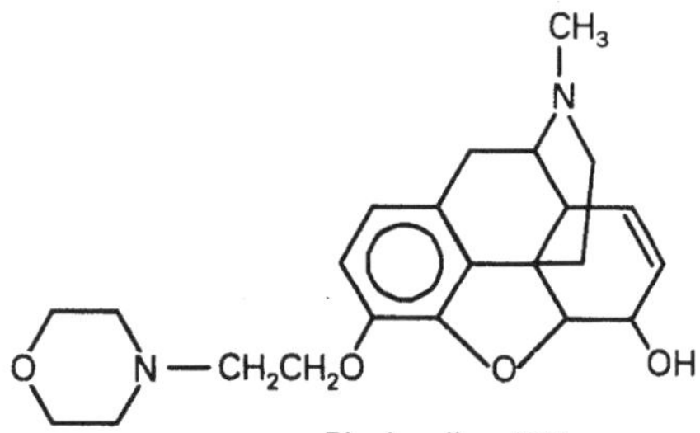

Pholcodine (95)

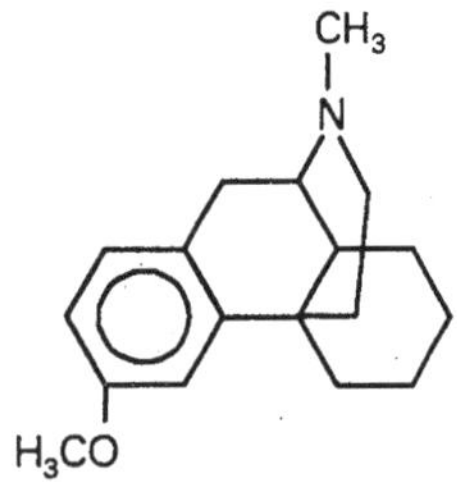

Dextromethorphan (96)

2.3.3.3 Antiparkinsonian drugs

Parkinson's disease was first described by James Parkinson in 1817. It is characterized by tremors, rigidity, and poverty of movement causing postural instability. The head and/or other parts of the body shake uninterruptedly. The treatment of this disease involves physiotherapy besides drugs, and requires psychological support. The drugs used for the treatment of this disease are known as antiparkinsonian drugs. They include Levodopa (97) and Carbidopa (98).

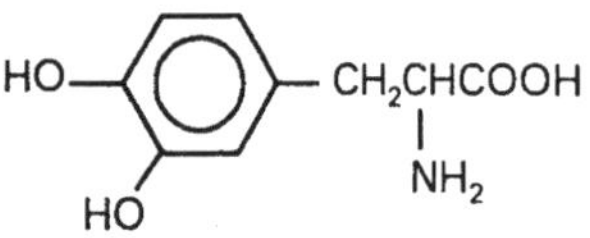

Levodopa (97)

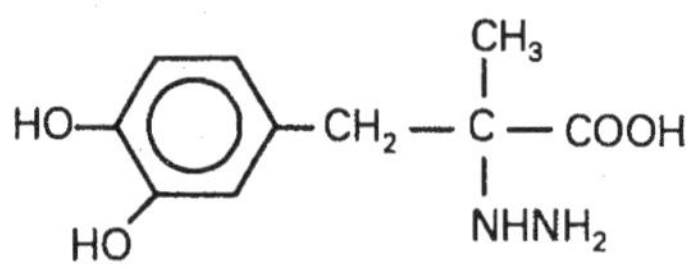

Carbidopa (98)

2.3.3.4 Neuroleptics

Neuroleptics or antipsychotics are drugs that counteract or minimize hallucinations and delusions, and facilitate social adjustment. While hallucinations consist of seeing an imaginary scene or hearing an imaginary sound as clearly as if they were really there, delusions are false belief which a person holds. Neuroleptics act on the brain. The notable drugs in this category are: (i) chlorpromazine (Thorazine) (99), (ii) haloperidol (Haldol) (100), (iii) loxapine (Loxitane), and (iv) molindone (Moban). These neuroleptics are used to treat all forms of schizophrenia, psychotic depression and mania.

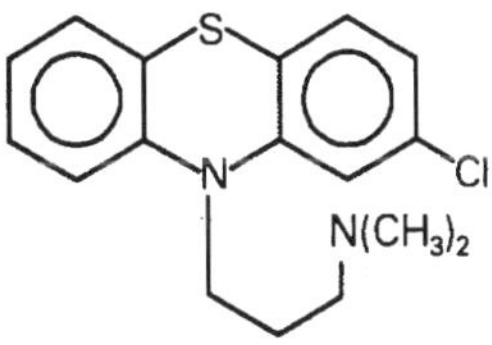

Chlorpromazine (99)
(Thorazine)

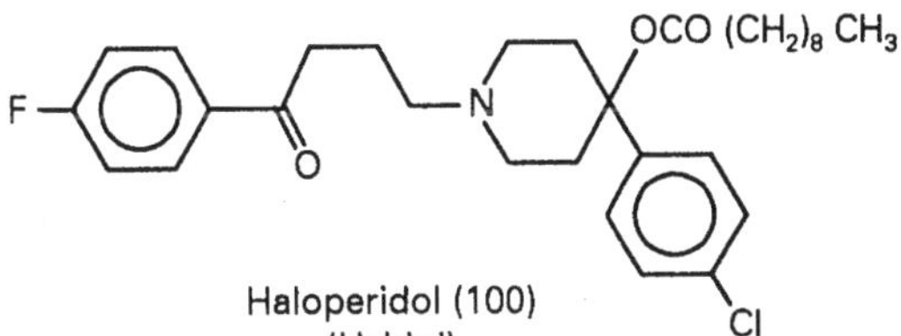

Haloperidol (100)
(Haldol)

2.4 *Drugs acting on the peripheral nervous system (PNS)*

While the central nervous system represents the brain and spinal cord, the peripheral nervous system comprises all parts of the nervous system lying outside the CNS. It includes the cranial nerves and spinal nerves and their branches which link the receptors and effector organs (muscles or glands) with the brain and spinal cord. The nerves are comprised of bundles of fibres which are used for transmitting the impulses of sensation, motion, information, etc., between the brain or spinal cord and other parts of the body. Certain chemicals, like adrenaline and acetylcholine, serve as neurotransmitters and play an important biochemical role inside the human body. The CNS is ultimately responsible for the integration of all nervous activities.

The peripheral nervous system (PNS) is composed of the somatic and autonomic nervous system (Fig. 2.8). The autonomic nervous system (ANS) supplies nerves to the heart, the smooth muscles, the glands and the viscera, and governs the functions of these organs. The ANS possesses inherent physiological activity. The interference with the ANS does not completely prevent its functions and thus it enjoys some degree of autonomy and that is the reason why it is called the autonomic nervous system. This is in contrast to the somatic nervous system (SNS), which is related to the non-reproductive parts of the body such as the skeletal muscles, which become totally defunct following the interruption of their motor nerves.

The ANS is subdivided into two groups, based on the chemical neurotransmitters that mediate autonomic nerve impulses. They are the parasympathetic nervous system and the sympathetic nervous system, which are usually in a state of dynamic equilibrium. Acetylcholine (101) is the chemical neurotransmitter in the parasympathetic division, and norepinephrine (102) is the principal chemical neurotransmitter in the sympathetic division. The sympathetic nervous system enables the individual to adjust to stress and strain, and prepares the body for 'flight or fight'. On the other hand, the parasympathetic nervous system is mainly associated with tissue-building reactions. A person can still survive after the complete elimination of the functions of the sympathetic nervous system, but not of the parasympathetic nervous system.

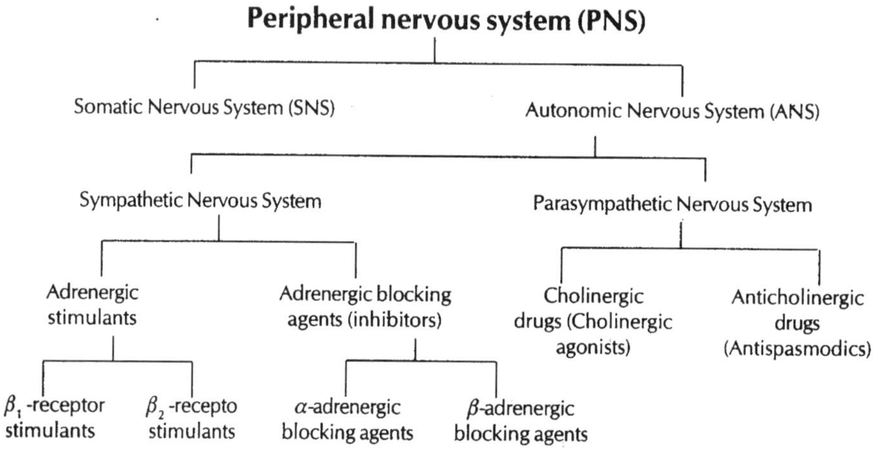

Fig. 2.8 *Classification of peripheral nervous system.*

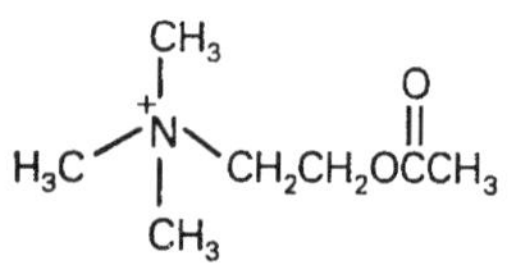

Acetylcholine (101)

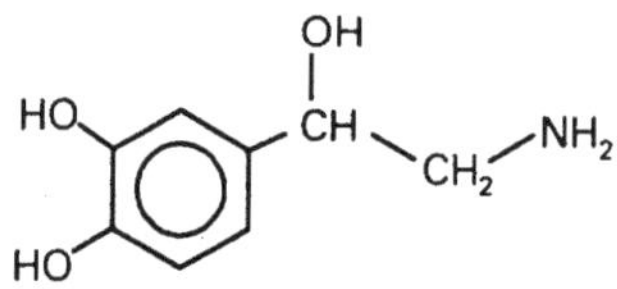

Norepinephrine (102)

2.4.1 Sympathetic nervous system

A drug that stimulates the sympathetic nervous system is called 'sympathomimetic'. The pharmacological actions of some of these drugs resemble endogenous compounds like adrenaline and related substances and come under this category. They are of two types: (i) Adrenergic stimulants, and (ii) Adrenergic blocking agents.

2.4.1.1 Adrenergic stimulants

The sympathetic nervous system is regulated by adrenergic drugs. At times of stress, the impulses of the sympathetic nerves release the chemical compounds, norepinephrine (102) and epinephrine (26) to the effector organs. *The drugs whose action is similar to that of norepinephrine and epinephrine are termed as adrenergic stimulants or agonists.* Epinephrine (26) was earlier termed as adrenaline. The most common adrenergic stimulants are norepinephrine (102), epinephrine (26), phenylephrine (103) and ephedrine (104).

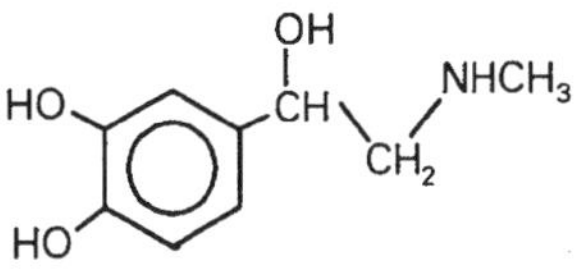

Epinephrine (26)
(adrenaline)

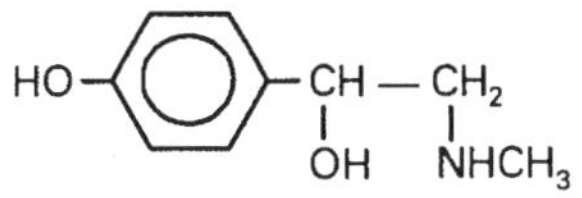

Phenylephrine (103)

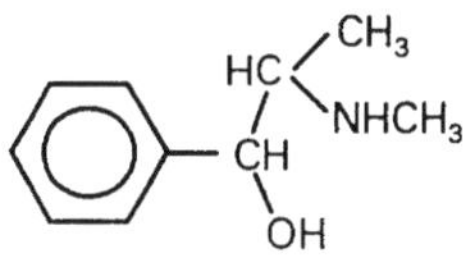

Ephedrine (104)

It has been reported that D (–) - epinephrine is about 20 times more active than the L(+) - epinephrine. Epinephrine is a secondary amine, whereas norepinephrine is a primary amine. It is found that the (–) isomer of norepinephrine is 27 times more potent than the (+) isomer. Norepinephrine raises blood pressure by peripheral vasoconstriction. There are two types of adrenergic stimulants: (i) β_1 - receptor stimulants, and (ii) β_2 - receptor stimulants.

β_1-receptor stimulants (agonists) Salbutamol (25) is an example. It is used as a bronchodilator. This property is more prominent than its effect on the heart.

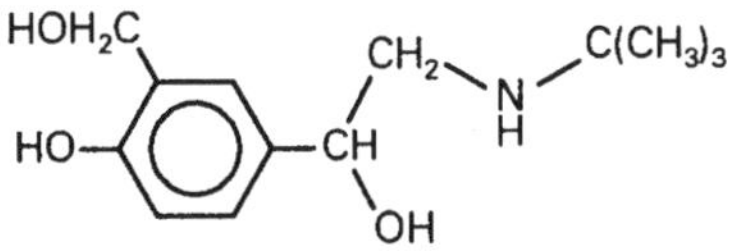

Salbutamol (25)
(Ventolin)

β_2-receptor stimulants (agonists) These drugs are very effective in relaxing the smooth muscles of the bronchi and uterus and, therefore, are used for relief in asthma and labour pains; e.g., terbutaline (Brethine) (105).

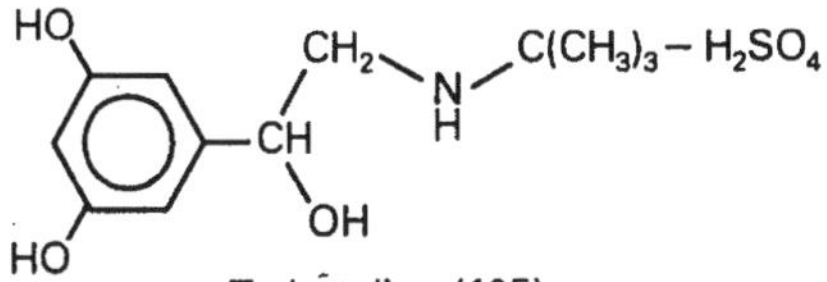

Terbutaline (105)
(Brethine)

2.4.1.2 Adrenergic blocking agents

They are of two types, i.e., alpha-adrenoceptor blocking agents and beta-adrenoceptor blocking agents. In tissues having both types of receptors, such as blood vessels, alpha stimulation causes contraction whereas beta stimulation causes relaxation. An α-adrenergic blocking drug in such a tissue causes vasodilation. In organs which have only beta-receptors, e.g., the heart, the β-blockers are found to oppose the excitory effect of norepinephrine, which is released from the nerve endings.

α-Adrenoceptor Blocking Agents (antagonists) They exert a vasodilatory effect causing a lowering of blood pressure, e.g., phenoxybenzamine (106) and ergotamine (23).

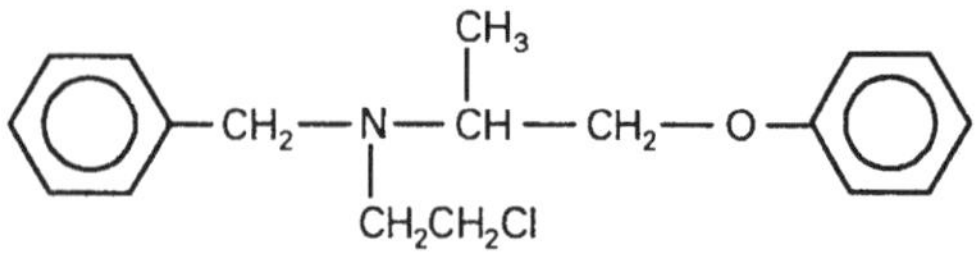

Phenoxybenzamine (106)

β-Adrenoceptor Blocking Agents (antagonists) They usually inhibit the action of catecholamines at the β-adrenergic receptor sites. These agents normally retard cardiac stress, and are used in the treatment of angina pectoris and cardiac arrhythmias. They are also used to control blood pressure, e.g., propranolol (107).

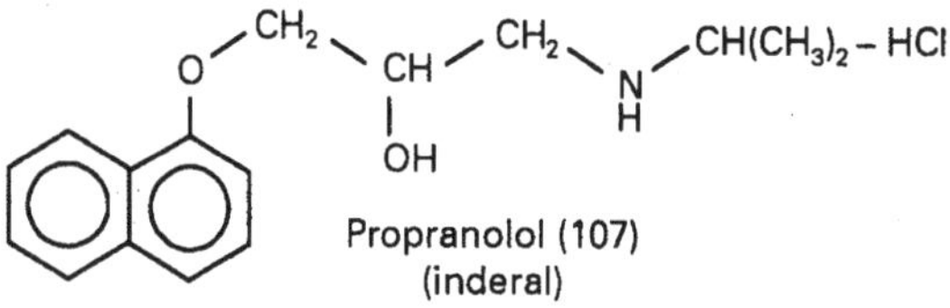

Propranolol (107)
(inderal)

2.4.2 Parasympathetic nervous system

The parasympathetic nervous system is regulated by cholinergic drugs. This is also referred to as cholinergic division and acetylcholine (101) is the chemical compound which mediates impulses between nerves. Acetylcholine produces the same effects as electrical stimulation of parasympathetic nerves. Drugs that stimulate the parasympathetic nervous system are called parasympathomimetic or cholinomimetic agents. Cholinergic agonists are cholinomimetic agents that act directly at receptor sites for acetylcholine (101). Drugs that block or inhibit the parasympathetic nervous system responses by possessing affinity, but without intrinsic activity for cholinergic receptors, are called cholinergic antagonists or parasympatholytic agents.

2.4.2.1 Cholinergic drugs

Cholinergic drugs include: (i) choline esters (carbachol (108), bethanechol (109)) which act at all sites like acetylcholine; (ii) alkaloids (pilocarpine (110), muscarine (111), arecoline) which act selectively on end organs that respond to acetylcholine; and (iii) cholinesterase inhibitors or anticholinesterases (physostigmine (112), neostigmine (113)) which inactivate the enzyme that destroys acetylcholine, allowing the chemical transmitter to persist and produce intensified effects.

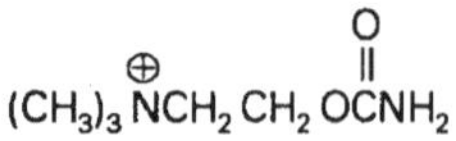

Carbachol (108)

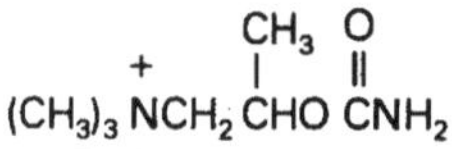

Bethanechol (109)

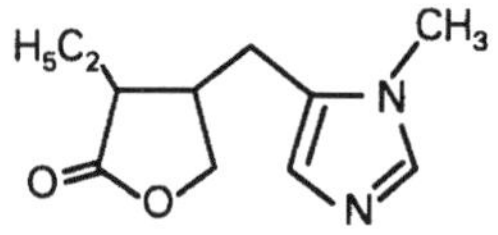

Pilocarpine (110)

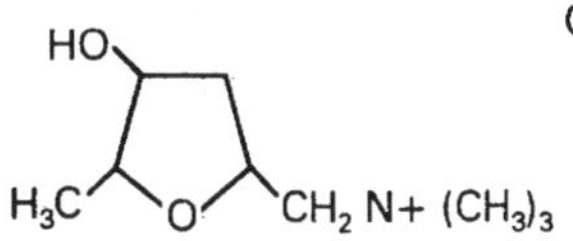

Muscarine (111)

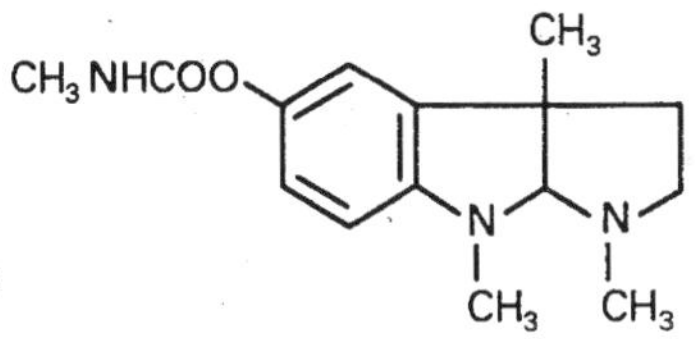

Physostigmine (112)

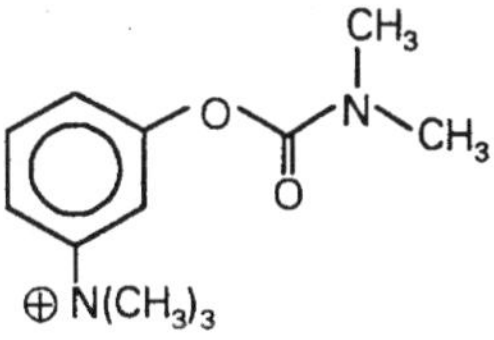

Neostigmine (113)

There are two types of cholinergic receptors. Muscarine receptors are those in which muscarine is the cholinergic agonist and nicotine is the cholinergic agonist at nicotine receptors. Acetylcholine is of great importance in the body, with a huge variety of effects, and is rapidly destroyed.

2.4.2.2 Anticholinergic drugs (Antispasmodic agents)

Anticholinergic drugs regulate abnormal muscular activity to normal levels by preventing acetylcholine from producing an excessive stimulatory effect. The violent contraction of the involuntary (smooth) muscles like the intestine, stomach, heart, blood vessels, etc., due to an excessive quantity of acetylcholine, is called a 'spasm'. This is the reason why the anticholinergic drugs are also called antispasmodic agents which are essentially antiacetylcholine in action. Atropine (114) acts by competing for the same receptors as acetylcholine, occupying them and thus rendering the acetylcholine ineffective. Generally, it is an acetylcholine receptor blocker. Papaverine (77) is also an important antispasmodic agent. The biological action of papaverine is musculotropic, while the biological action of atropine is neurotropic. Diphenhydramine (50) is twice as powerful as papaverine as an antispasmodic agent.

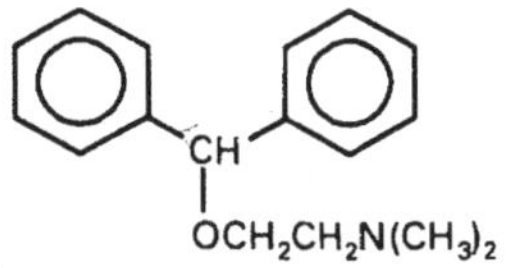

Diphenhydramine (50)
(Benadryl)

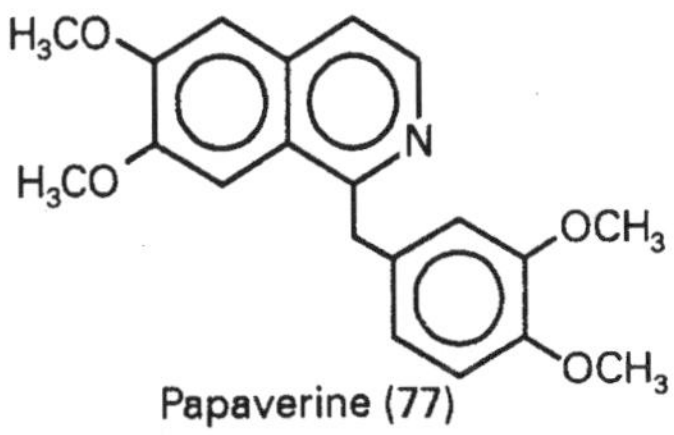

Papaverine (77)

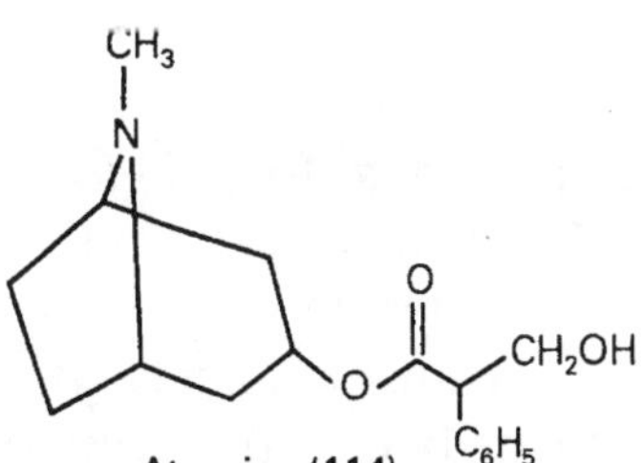

Atropine (114)

2.5 *Drugs acting on the cardiovascular system*

Cardiovascular drugs are those drugs which act on the heart or blood vessels. The human heart is an important organ, similar to a mechanical pump, that distributes the blood to all the cells, tissues and organs of the body. The heart consists of four chambers: the upper chambers are called the atria and the lower chambers, the ventricles. That is, the heart has right and left atria and right and left ventricles. The atria have openings into their corresponding ventricles with one-way valves. The ventricles are muscular and thick-walled while the atria are relatively thin-walled. Even among the ventricles, the walls of the left ventricle are 3 to 4 times thicker than that of the right ventricle and, because of this, it pumps the blood to the entire body through the aorta. The right ventricle pumps blood to the lungs through the pulmonary artery. The heart also contributes to the elimination of unwanted products and toxic materials from the same tissues and organs.

Most diseases of the heart are caused by: (i) congenital structural defects, (ii) reduced blood supply to the heart, (iii) rate and rhythm of contraction, (iv) decreased efficiency of the heart muscle, and (v) localized infections. Cardiovascular drugs may be broadly classified into the following types.

i) Antihypertensive drugs
ii) Anti-arrhythmic drugs
iii) Cardiotonic drugs
iv) Vasodilators
v) Antihypercholesterolemic drugs

2.5.1 Antihypertensive drugs

Hypertension is a common disease from which many people suffer. The terms *hypertension* refer to high blood pressure and *hypotension* to low blood pressure. *Hypertension has been defined, according to the World Health Organisation (WHO), as a measurement of the systolic (contraction of the heart) blood pressure in excess of 140 mm Hg and diastolic (expansion of the heart) blood pressure exceeding 90 mm Hg. The normal adult should have a systolic pressure equal to or below 140 mm Hg together with a diastolic pressure equal to or below 90 mm Hg.* Blood pressure is measured with an instrument called a 'sphygmomanometer'. The exact cause of hypertension is unknown, but we do know that hypertension is the result of defects in the haemodynamic and biochemical functions of the body. The conditions leading to hypertension include obesity, increased salt intake, excessive use of alcohol, cigarette smoking, atherosclerotic complications, and those associated with pregnancy. The small arterioles used for transporting blood from the arteries to the tissue capillaries, and veins carrying blood to the heart get excessive stimulation due to the sympathetic nervous system. This results in arteriole contraction and increased resistance to the flow of blood. As a result, the blood pressure increases. The other causes for elevated B.P. are tension and emotional stress, which lead to the increased production of octapeptide Angiotensin-II (see page 26). Any medicine used for counteracting this condition of reducing blood pressure and its accompanying symptoms, is known as an antihypertensive or hypotensive drug. An ideal antihypertensive drug should reduce blood pressure through vasodilation, without any side effects or development of tolerance through continuous usage. The drug should be administrable orally. The classification and follow-up of blood pressure measurements according to "The Fifth Report of the Joint National Committee on Detection, Education, and Treatment of High Blood Pressure (JNC-V), USA, 1993" is given in Table 2.7.

Table 2.7 *Follow-up of Blood Pressure Measurements*

Category	**Systolic Blood Pressure (mm Hg)**	**Diastolic Blood Pressure (mm Hg)**	**Follow-up Recommended**
Normal	<130	<85	Recheck in 2 years
High Normal	130–139	85–89	Recheck in 1 year
Hypertension			
Stage-1 (mild)	140–159	90–99	Confirm within 2 months
Stage-2 (moderate)	160–179	100–109	Refer within 1 month
Stage-3 (severe)	180–209	110–119	Refer within 1 week
Stage-4 (very severe)	≥ 210	≥ 120	Refer immediately

The antihypertensive drugs include the following four categories. They are:

(i) ACE inhibitors; captopril (capoten) (13), enalapril (vasotec) (30), ramipril (altace);

(ii) Calcium channel blockers; nifedipine (115), diltiazem (cardizem SR or CD) (116), amlodipine, felodipine (plendil) (117);

(iii) β-blockers; propranolol (inderal) (107), atenolol (sectral) (118);

(iv) Diuretics; furosemide (lasix), bumetanide (bumex), and metolazone (diulo)) (119).

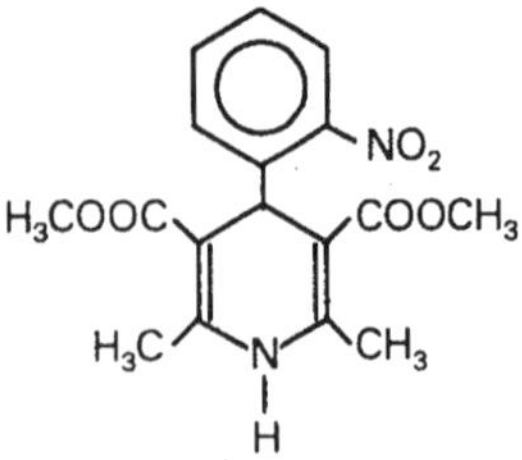

Nifedipine (115)

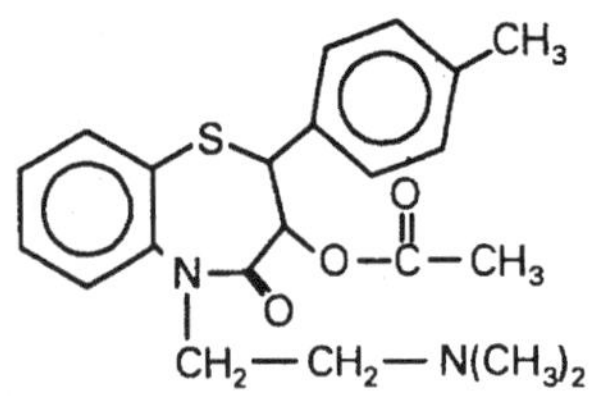

Diltiazem (116)

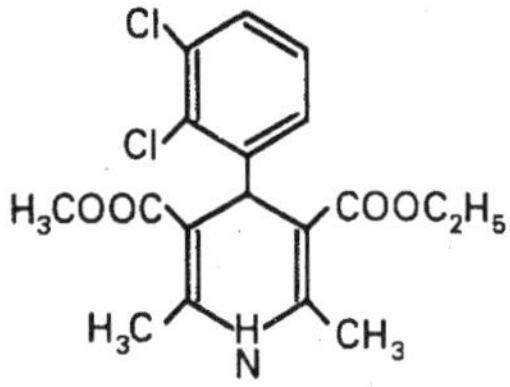

Felodipine (117)
(Plendil)

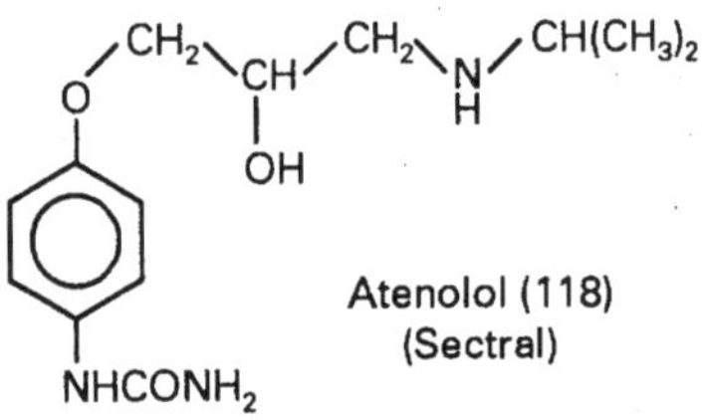

Atenolol (118)
(Sectral)

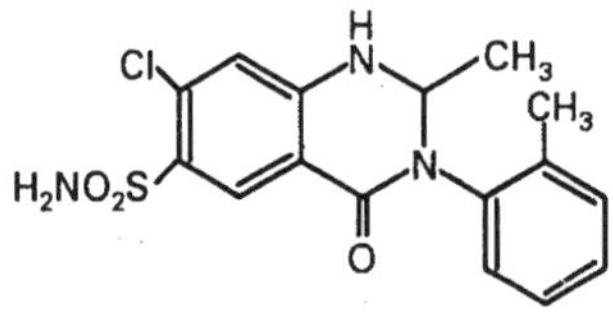

Metolazone (119)
(diulo)

2.5.2 Anti-arrythmic drugs

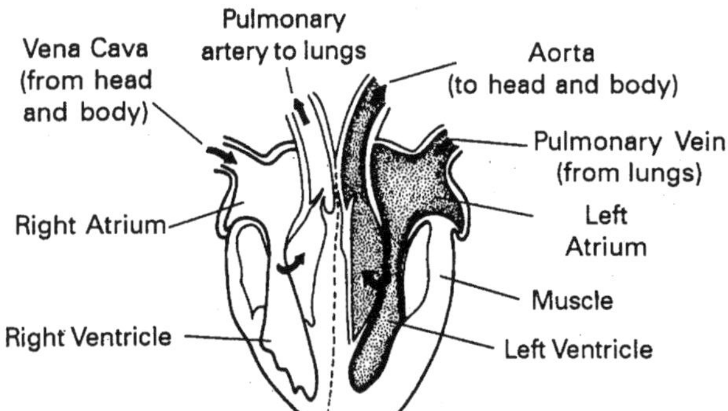

Fig. 2.9 *Structure of the heart.*

Arrythmia is defined *as an abnormal rhythm (beat) of the heart*. When the rate of the heart is inordinately slowed down or greatly accelerated, its efficiency decreases, and it may not be in a position to pump the necessary amount of blood. Arrythmia is an alteration in the normal sequence of electrical impulse activation, that leads to the contraction of the myocardium. It is manifested as an abnormality either in the rate, in the site from which the impulses originate, or in the conduction through the myocardium. Many factors influence the normal rhythm of electrical activity in the heart (Fig. 2.9). Diseases such as atherosclerosis, hyperthyroidism, or lung disease may also cause arrythmia. The commonly used drugs include: Quinidine (Cardioquin, Duraquin, Quinora), Procainamide (Procan, Promine, Pronestyl, Rhythmin) (120),

Lidocaine (Xylocaine, Lidopen) (121), Tocainide (Tonocard), and Mexiletine (Mexitil) (122).

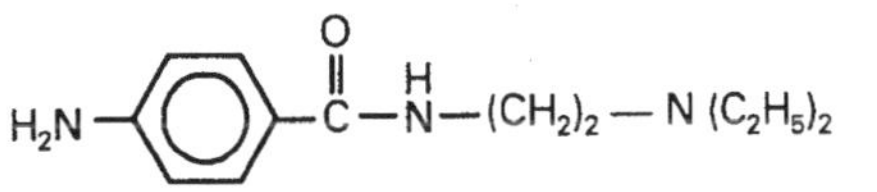

Procainamide (120)
(Pronestyl)

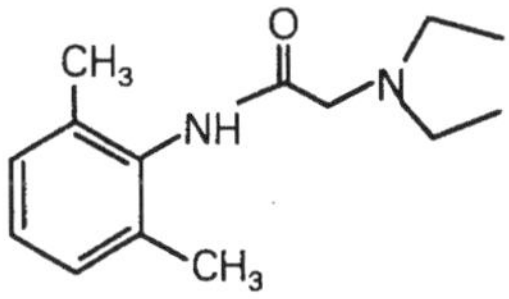

Lidocaine (121)
(Xylocaine, Lidopen)

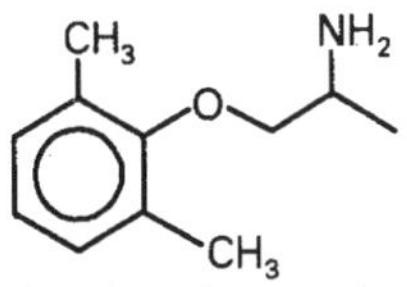

Mexiletine (122)
(Mexitil)

2.5.3 Cardiotonic drugs

Cardiotonic agents increase the force of myocardial contractions, without any corresponding increase in oxygen consumption. The heart becomes a more efficient pump to circulate the blood to different parts of the body. Cardiac glycosides are an important class of naturally-occuring drugs, used as cardiotonic agents, and are effective on the heart. Cardiotonic drugs are particularly useful in the treatment of congestive heart failure and associated oedema. Cardiac glycosides occur mainly in plants and, in rare cases, in animals like the poisonous toads. *Digitalis purpurea* or the foxglove plant, *Digitalis lanata, Strophanthus gratus*, and *Strophanthus kombe* are the major plant sources of cardiac glycosides. Digitalis, digitoxin, digoxin (21), and ouabain are the most commonly used cardiac glycosides obtained from the above plants.

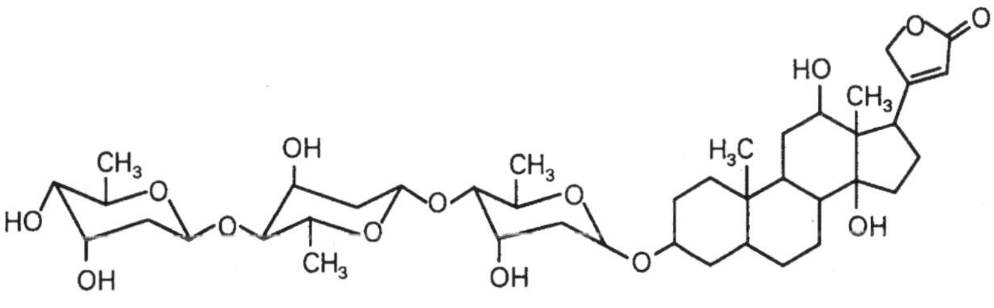

Digoxin (21)

2.5.4 Vasodilators

The coronary artery is the supply route of blood carrying oxygen from the left ventricle to all the heart tissues, including the ventricles themselves. When the coronary artery becomes less efficient in supplying blood and oxygen to the heart, the heart is said to be *ischaemic* (short of oxygen). *Angina pectoris* is the disease of the coronary artery. Angina is the primary symptom of ischemic heart disease, characterized by a sudden, severe pain originating in the chest, often radiating to the left shoulder and down the left arm. This is known as a heart attack. Chest pain is one of the symptoms of heart attack. Typical angina, usually, is the result of an advanced state of atherosclerosis. Angina is generally felt after unaccustomed exercise, large meals and stress.

The therapy for angina is directed at reducing and preventing anginal attacks by dialating the coronary artery. An ideal vasodilator drug should increase the blood flow without increasing the work of the heart. The various vasodilators are Nitroglycerin (22), Amyl nitrite, Diltiazem (Cardizem, Dilzem), and Cardene (116).

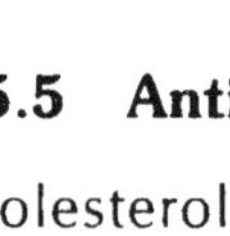

Nitroglycerin (22)
(Glonoin)

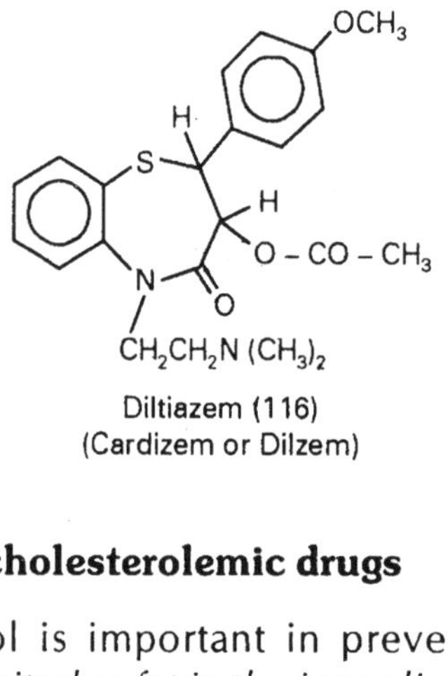

Diltiazem (116)
(Cardizem or Dilzem)

2.5.5 Antihypercholesterolemic drugs

Cholesterol control is important in preventing cardiac diseases. *Cholesterol is deposited as fat in the inner linings of arteries in human beings, resulting in atherosclerosis.* This may interfere with the supply of blood and cause high blood pressure and heart attacks. The range of serum cholesterol in normal individuals is 190–250 mg/dL, with approximately 30% in the free state and 70% as cholesterol esters. Reducing the absorption of cholesterol, increasing the metabolism, the biliary excretion of cholesterol and preventing the synthesis of cholesterol in the liver all help to avoid cardiac disorders. The decrease of fat content in the diet also brings down the cholesterol in the body. The use of unsaturated fats from vegetable sources appears to lead to decreased serum cholesterol. The various drugs used for controlling the cholesterol level are lovastatin (123), pravastatin (124), chlorfibrate (atromid-s), etc.

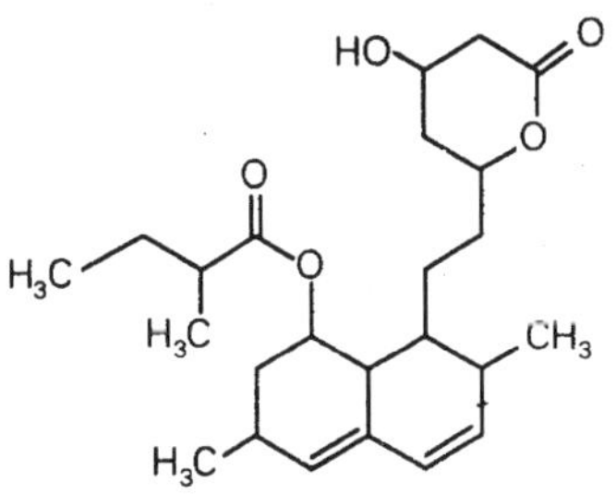

Lovastatin (123)

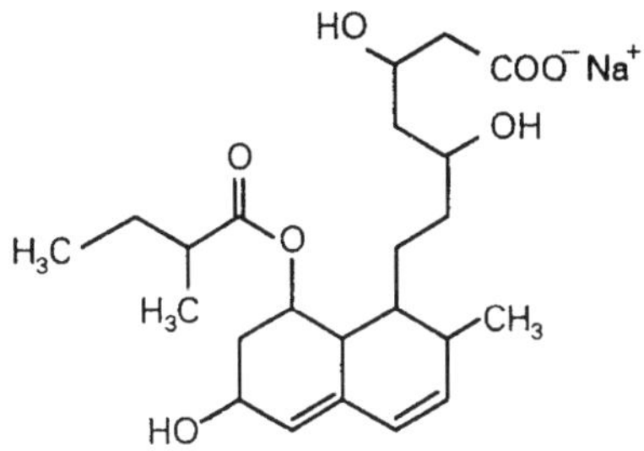

Pravastatin (124)

2.6 *Drugs acting on the hematopoietic system*

Hematopoiesis is the complex series of events that occur in the blood, which are involved in the formation, proliferation, differentiation and activation of red blood cells (erythrocytes), white blood cells (leucocytes) and platelets (thrombocytes). All blood cells originate within the bone marrow from a single class of pluripotent stem cells.

Blood is heavier, thicker and more viscous than water. The temperature of blood is about 38° C (100.4° F), which is slightly higher than normal body temperature.The pH of blood is about 7.40 (normal range: 7.35 to 7.45) (alkaline). Blood constitutes about 8% of the total body weight. The blood volume is 5 to 6 litres in an average-sized male and 4 to 5 litres in an average-sized female. Whole blood is composed of two portions: 55% blood is plasma, a watery liquid containing dissolved substances, and 45% is made up of cells and cell fragments. Plasma or blood plasma contains about 91.5% water and (7%) proteins. The proteins confined to blood are called plasma proteins. The various components of blood are given in Fig. 2.10.

Blood has three general functions: 1) transportation, 2) regulation, and 3) protection.

1) Transportation: Blood transports oxygen from the lungs to the cells of the body and CO_2 from the cells to the lungs. It also carries nutrients from the gastrointestinal tract to the cells, and metabolic waste products enter the blood from cells and hormones from endocrine glands to other body cells.

2) Regulation: Blood regulates its pH through buffers. It also adjusts the body temperature through the heat-absorbing and coolant properties of its water content and its variable rate of flow through the skin, where excess heat can be lost to the environment.

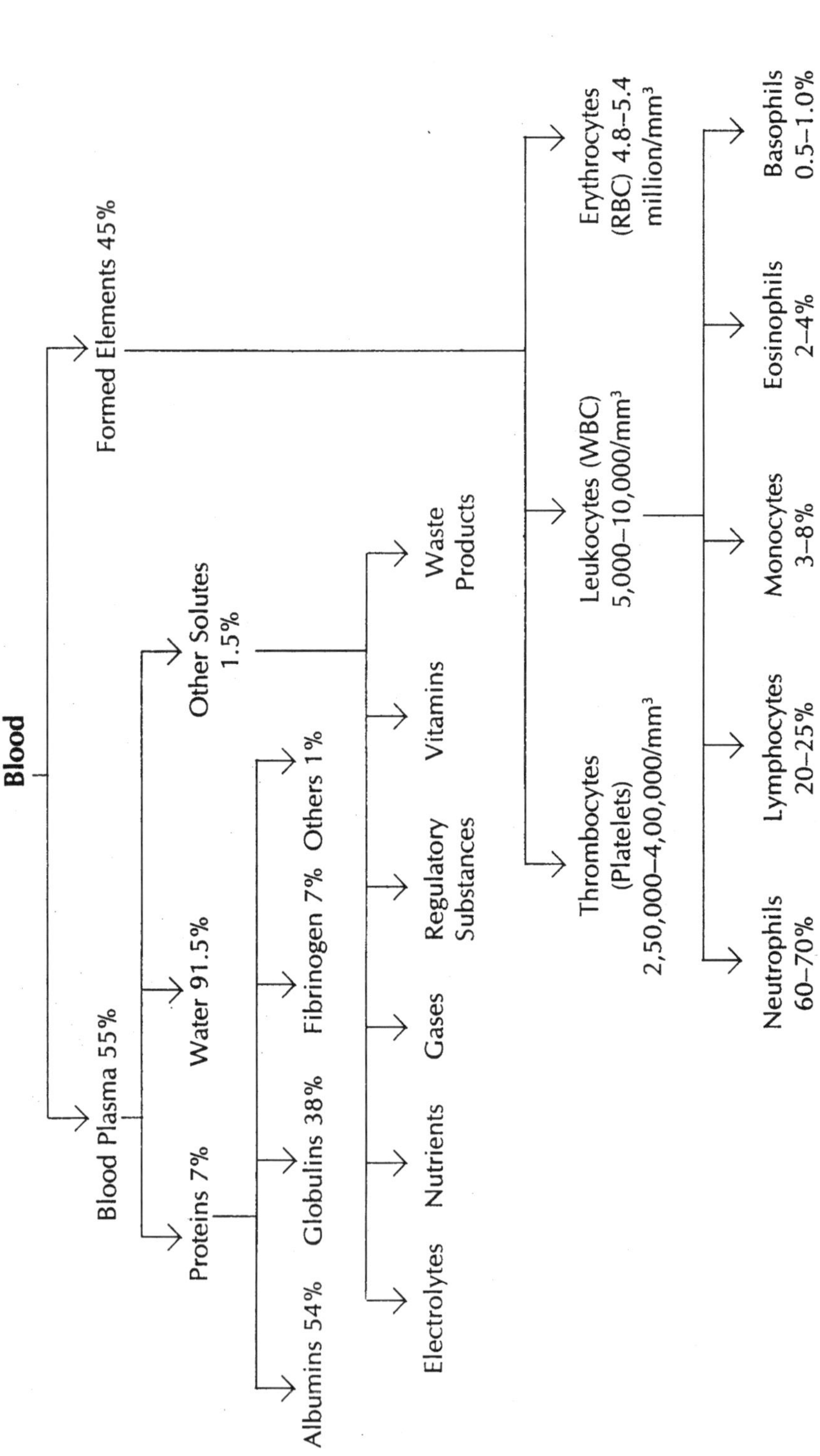

Fig. 2.10 *Composition of blood.*

3) Protection: The clotting mechanism protects against blood loss and certain phagocytic WBC or specialized plasma proteins, such as antibodies and interferon, protect against foreign microbes and toxins.

Among the drugs which act on the blood and the blood-forming organs, (i) anticoagulant and coagulant drugs, and (ii) anti-anemic drugs are very important.

2.6.1 Anticoagulant and coagulant drugs

Blood clotting involves a sequence of pathological actions. The human body has the remarkable ability to arrange either for clotting or to prevent clotting, whichever is required under pathogenic conditions. The clotting or coagulation of blood chokes the circulation of blood, leading to complications and even death. At the same time, the clotting of blood is also an important defensive mechanism which prevents excessive blood loss in case of an injury. The clotting of blood is called thrombosis, and the escape of blood from a ruptured blood vessel externally or internally is called hemorrhage.

Before studying the anticoagulant and coagulant drugs used in health care, it is necessary to know about blood clotting which is essentially a biochemical process. The mechanism of the coagulation scheme was explained by Morawitz in 1903. When an injury to a blood vessel or tissue occurs, an immediate vasoconstrictive reflex reduces the volume of blood flow and platelets begin to adhere to the injured cells, this is called *platelet adhesion*. The platelets subsequently release adenosine diphosphate (ADP) and prostaglandin endoperoxides that adhere to one another, forming a platelet plug. This is referred to as *platelet aggregation*, which leads to blood clotting. It is the fibrin which coagulates the blood. The mechanism of clot formation involves two reactions:

(i) Prothrombin + Ca^{2+} + Thromboplastin → Thrombin
(ii) Thrombin + Fibrinogen → Fibrin

Prothrombin which is formed in the liver reacts with thromboplastin that is released from injured tissue cells and from blood platelets, in the presence of calcium ions, to form thrombin. This thrombin converts fibrinogen (another protein formed in the liver) to fibrin, which results in a blood clot. Vitamin K is required for the biosynthesis of prothrombin in the liver which, in turn, binds to calcium ions and thromboplastin during its conversion to thrombin.

2.6.1.1 Anticoagulant drugs

Anticoagulants are drugs which prevent or prolong the coagulation time of blood. This can be achieved either by supressing the factors needed for coagulation or by stimulating the normal anticoagulants in the body. The important anticoagulants include heparin, coumarin derivatives, and sodium citrate.

Heparin Heparin (125), a mucopolysaccharide, was first used as anticoagulant in 1937. It occurs in most cells of the vascular system and in many tissues of the body including the liver, with an abundant supply from the lungs. Today, heparin is produced commercially by selective processing of pig intestines. Heparin is administered parenterally, as it is ineffective orally and its action is rapid but of short duration. It is generally given to post-operative patients and to those with acute infarctions (blood clottings), requiring immediate anticoagulant activity.

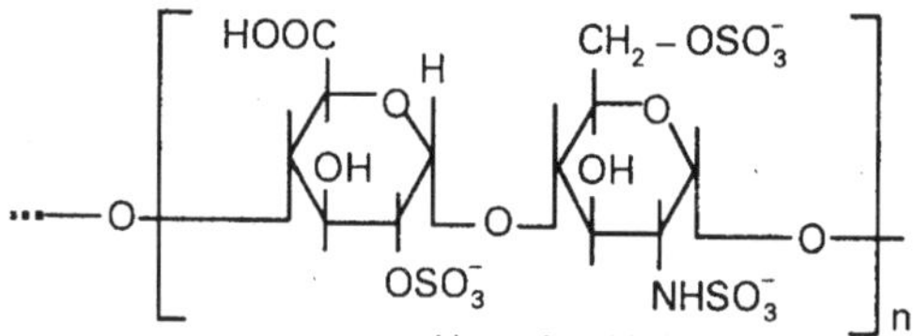

Heparin (125)

Coumarin and indanedione derivatives Coumarin derivatives are orally active anticoagulant drugs. Coumarins exert their effects *in vivo* only after a latent period of 12 to 48 hours. Their effect lasts for 1.5 to 5 days.

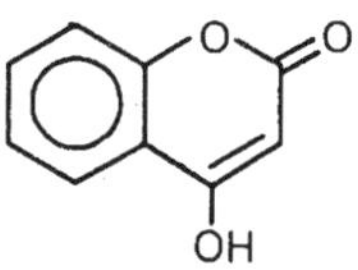

4-Hydroxycoumarin (126)

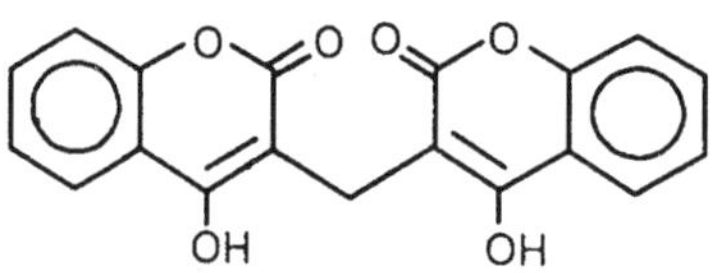

Bishydroxycoumarin (127)
(Dicumarol)

Some of the coumarin derivatives are: 4-hydroxycoumarin (126), Bishydroxycoumarin (dicumarol) (127), and warfarin sodium (128) which serve as anticoagulants. Warfarin is marketed as the sodium salt; 1,3-indandiones (anisidione) (129) are also anticoagulant drugs.

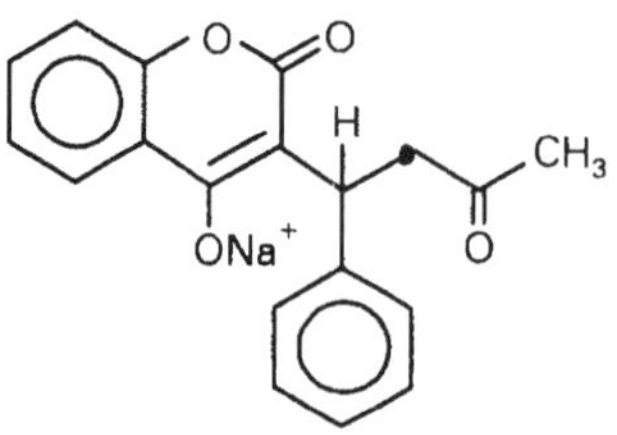

Warfarin sodium (128)

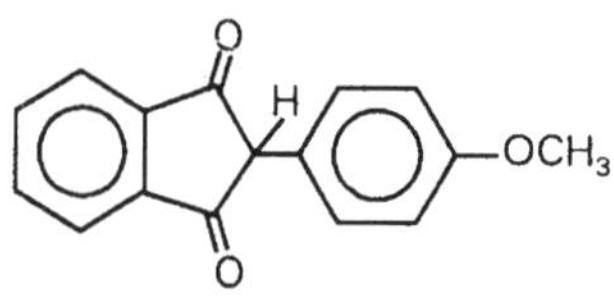

(129)
2-(p-methoxyphenyl)-
1,3-indandione (129)
(Anisidione, Miradon)

Sodium citrate Citric acid (130) is a water-soluble tricarboxylic acid, widely distributed in plants and in animal tissues and fluids. Citric acid (130) has many industrial and pharmaceutical uses, mostly (as an acidulant) in beverages, confectionaries, syrups, elixirs and tablets. Medicinally, citric acid is usually used as sodium citrate (trisodium citrate) (131) to serve as an *in vitro* anticoagulant. The citrate anion forms a soluble complex with calcium (132) (Fig. 2.11). By removing the calcium ion, one of the agents required to convert prothrombin to thrombin, i.e., clot formation, is inhibited.

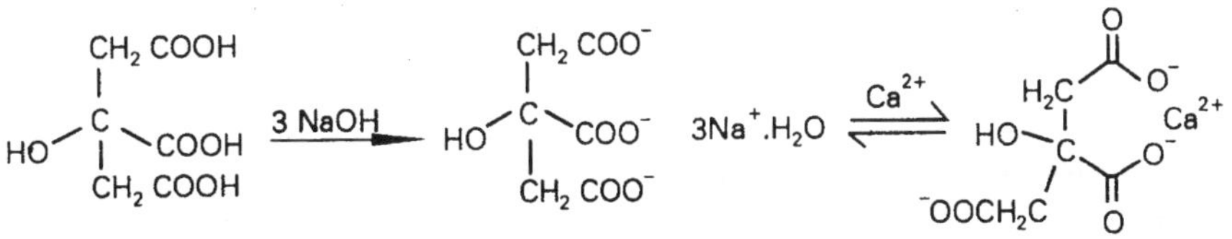

Citric acid (130) Trisodium citrate (131) Calcium citrate (132)

Fig. 2.11 *Formation of calcium citrate.*

2.6.1.2 Coagulant drugs

Drugs that are useful for the clotting of blood are called coagulants. Generally, coagulants include vitamin K and its analogs, proteins and amino acids, and plasma coagulants.

Vitamin K In 1929, a Danish scientist, Dam, found that the deficiency of vitamin K increases the blood clotting time. Vitamin K refers to a

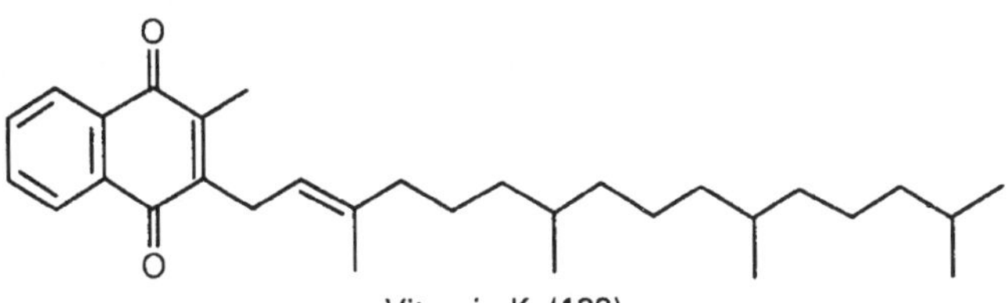

Vitamin K_1 (133)

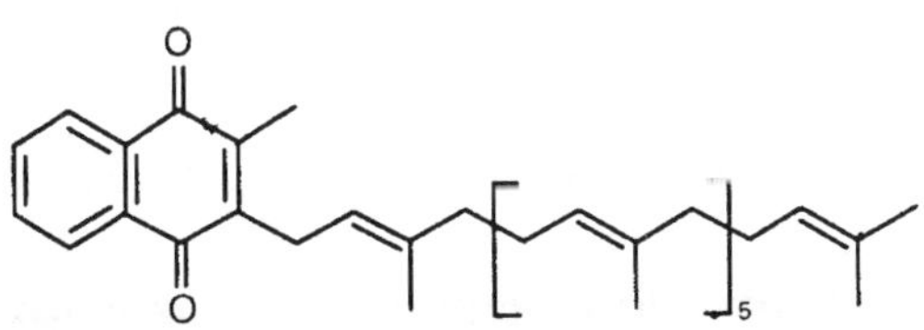

Vitamin K_2 (134)

coagulation vitamin. The deficiency is characterized by an increase in blood clotting time. This is the result of the impaired synthesis of prothrombin and other proteins required for blood clotting. In normal adults, the need for vitamin K is met by diet, in which leafy green vegetables are an excellent source. Vitamin K_1 (133) and vitamin K_2 (134), which differ only in the structure of their side chains, possess the same coagulant properties (see Chapter 3). Vitamin K_1 is also known as phylloquinone.

Proteins and amino acids Proteins such as thrombin, fibrinogen and gelatin, and aminocaproic acid (an amino acid) are used systemically or topically for their coagulating effects. Thrombin, fibrin and gelatin are used topically to clot oozing blood. Fibrin and thrombin play an important role in the clotting process, as described earlier. In addition to promoting clotting, these proteins may mechanically aid platelets in stopping bleeding.

2.6.2 Anti-anemic drugs

In a normal person's body, there is a balance between the formation and destruction of red blood cells. Any disease may upset this delicate balance and decrease the production or increase the wastage. *Anemia may be defined as a state in which the level of haemoglobin in the blood is less than what is required.* Haemoglobin is a complex molecule, a combination of "haem" (a red pigment) and "globin" (protein). Haemoglobin provides the oxygen-transport mechanism for the blood. The clinical features of anemia reflect the diminished oxygen-carrying capacity of the blood. Iron is essential for haemoglobin synthesis. Most anemias are deficiency diseases, caused by insufficient concentrations of iron, vitamin B_{12} or folic acid.

Iron Iron deficiency is the most common cause of anemia. The human body contains about 2–6 gm of iron (male: 50 mg/kg, female: 35 mg/kg). About two-thirds of the total iron content in the human body is present in haemoglobin. A normal person absorbs up to 10% iron through his/her diet (1–4 mg/day). The total iron loss per day is about 0.5–1 mg, and the menstrual loss is about 30 mg/period. A pregnant woman needs nearly 2.5 mg extra iron per day for the foetus, placenta and normal blood loss at the time of delivery. Iron deficiency can be overcome by treatment with ferrous sulphate ($FeSO_4.7H_2O$) tablets, which is very effective. Ferrous fumarate tablets, ferrous succinate and ferrous glycine sulphate are the other alternatives.

Vitamin B_{12} Vitamin B_{12}, known as cyanocobalamin, is a red, cobalt-containing substance. The molecule has a modified porphyrin unit (a class that includes the "haem" of haemoglobin and the chlorophyll of plants) coordinating a trivalent cobalt ion. Vitamin B_{12} has been isolated from the liver and from fermented liquors of *Streptomyces griseus* and certain other microorganisms; it is also present in cow's milk. Vitamin B_{12} deficiency causes pernicious anemia. Pernicious anemia is the result of failure of the bone-marrow to produce normal, new blood cells. Vitamin B_{12} is used to counter this condition (for structure, see page 131).

Folic acid Folic acid (pteroylglutamic acid) (135) deficiency causes macrocytic anemias, a condition in whch the level of blood platelets and polynuclear erythrocytes is decreased, accompanied by gastrointestinal disturbances. The daily requirement of this vitamin is estimated at 0.5 mg and foods such as spinach, asparagus, bananas, strawberries, bone-marrow, liver and kidney are good dietary sources.

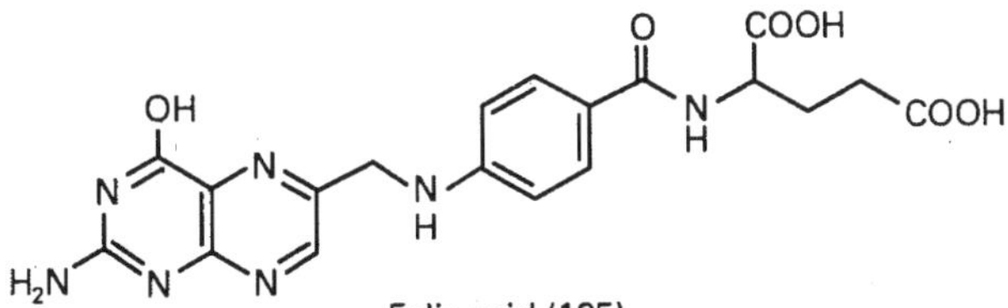

Folic acid (135)

2.7 *Drugs acting on the renal system*

The renal system refers to a mechanism relating to the kidneys. Drugs acting on the kidneys are broadly classified as diuretics and antidiuretics. Diuretics are chemicals that increase the rate of urine formation. The use of diuretic leads to the increased excretion of electrolytes, such as Na^+ Cl^- and water, from the body. Water constitutes the major portion of the human body mass. In an average adult male and female 60 and 51 per cent, respectively, of body mass is water. The primary target organ for diuretics is the kidney. The important functions of the kidney are: (i) to maintain a homeostatic balance of electrolytes and water (homeostatics is a physiological process by which the internal systems of the body such as blood pressure, body temperature, acid-base balance, are maintained at an equilibrium, despite variations in the external conditions) and, (ii) to excrete the water-soluble end products of metabolism. The kidney accomplishes these functions through the formation of urine by the nephrons (Fig. 2.12).

2.7.1 Nephron

Each kidney contains approximately one million nephrons and is capable of forming urine independently. The nephrons are composed of a bunch of capillary vessels called the glomerulus, which is enclosed in Bowman's capsule, and a long tubule which is functionally and anatomically divided into three parts—(i) the proximal tubule, (ii) the loop of Henle, and (iii) the distal tubule. Each compartment of the nephron contributes to the normal functioning of the kidney.

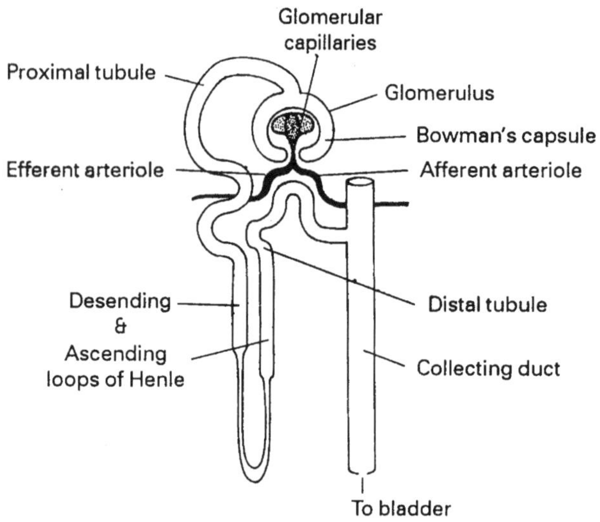

Fig. 2.12 *The structure of a nephron.*

The nephron also consists of a collecting tubule which leads to the bladder where the urine is stored. Each day, the body produces about 200 litres of glomerular filtrate which is modified during its passage in the renal tubules as 1.5 litres of urine, and the rest is reabsorbed. Urine formation begins with the filtration of blood at the glomerulus. Approximately 1200 ml of blood per minute flows through both the kidneys and reaches the nephron through afferent arterioles under high capillary pressure. The process of glomerular filtration results in the excretion of numerous end products of metabolism. They contain not only the waste products but also the essential constitutents of the extracellular fluid such as water, electrolytes, and nutrients. These must be reabsorbed to maintain the volume and the composition of the extracellular fluid. The homeostatic function of the kidney necessitates the reabsorption of most of the ingredients of the filtrate. The fluid within the cell (intracellular) is in osmotic equilibrium with the extracellular fluid. The changes in the extracellular fluid composition lead to changes in the intracellular fluid composition and function. The extracellular fluid composition is also influenced by changes in kidney function. Sodium is filtered at the glomerulus and is reabsorbed at the proximal tubule. About 85% of filtered bicarbonate is reabsorbed in the proximal tubule, which is one reason why urine is slightly acidic. Carbonic anhydrase (an enzyme) in proximal tubular epithelial cells catalyzes the generation of H_2CO_3, which dissociates to H^+ and HCO_3^-. The H^+ is passed on into the tubular fluid in exchange for Na^+ which enters the cells as $NaHCO_3$. On the whole, 65% of the filtered sodium is reabsorbed and goes back into the blood.

A change in the glomerular filtration rate or a defect in the tubular reabsorption disturbs the kidney function, resulting in an abnormal increase in the volume of extracellular fluid in the tissues and causing a condition known as 'oedema'. Oedema is also caused by congestive heart failure, nephritis, hepatic cirrhosis and ascites, and premenstrual tension. Diuretics are mainly used to increase the excretion of sodium chloride and water. The extra electrolytes, urea, uric acid and other substances that are rejected by the body are excreted in the form of urine. Diuretics are very effective in the treatment of cardiac oedema, especially the one related with congestive heart failure. Diuretics are used extensively in various type of disorders, e.g. (i) nephrotic syndrome, (ii) diabetes insipidus, (iii) nutritional oedema, (iv) cirrhosis of the liver, (v) hypertension, (vi) oedema of pregnancy, and (vii) to lower intraocular and cerebrospinal fluid pressure. Diuretic drugs can be broadly categorized into 5 groups (Fig. 2.13).

Diuretic drugs

Purine or Xanthine diuretics	Aldosterone inhibitors	High-ceiling or Loop diuretics	Carbonic anhydrase inhibitors	Thiazide diuretics

Fig. 2.13 *The classification of diuretic drugs.*

2.7.2 Purine or xanthine diuretics

These are structural analogues of purine and xanthine. Caffeine (78), theophylline (136) and theobromine (137) are the three important members of the xanthine diuretics which are found commonly in coffee, tea, cocoa, etc. These compounds are weak diuretics which act by inhibiting absorption of sodium chloride and water in the renal tubules.

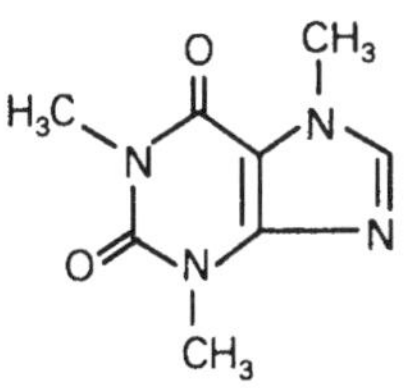

Caffeine (78)

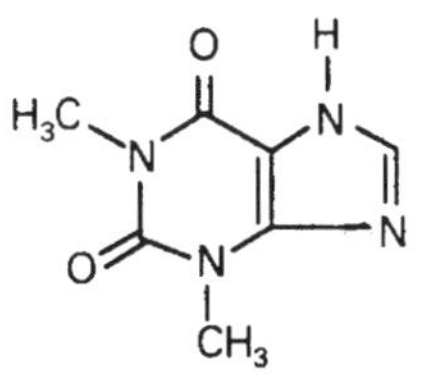

Theophylline (136)

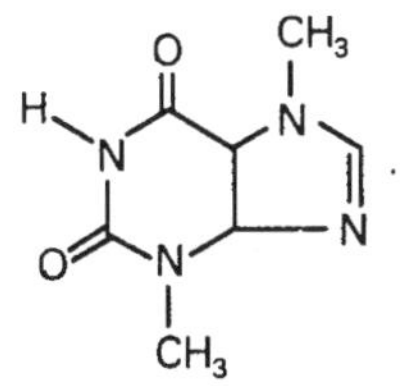

Theobromine (137)

2.7.3 Aldosterone inhibitors

Aldosterone, a naturally-occuring hormone secreted by the adrenal cortex, promotes the reabsorption and retention of Na^+, Cl^- and water in the distal tubule. A substance that inhibits the action of aldosterone could be a good diuretic drug. Spironolactone (138) and metyrapone (139) are the two prominent diuretic agents of this group. They belong to the corticosteroid group. Spironolactone binds to the aldosterone receptor preventing aldosterone from binding to its receptor. Therefore, aldosterone cannot cause the reabsorption of Na^+, Cl^- and water.

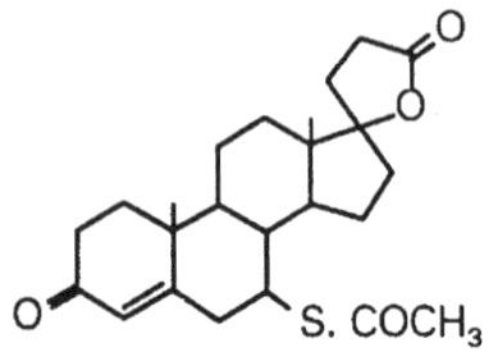

Spironolactone (138)

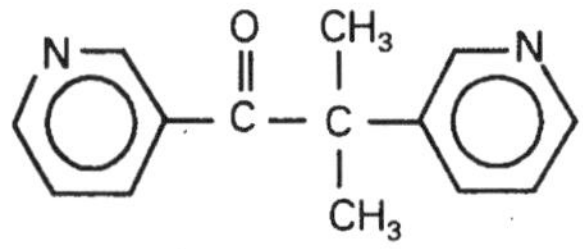

Metyrapone (139)

2.7.4 High-ceiling diuretics or loop diuretics

High-ceiling diuretics act mainly on the 'loop of Henle', for a relatively short duration (4 to 6 hrs), and essentially contain the carboxylic acid group. These diuretics have a greater effect than other commonly used diuretics and, hence, are called high-ceiling diuretics. They are also called loop diuretics. They cause a loss of Cl^-, Na^+ and K^+ ions. Bumetanide (140) and furosemide (141) are important drugs of this class. Bumetanide is particularly used in forced diuresis in conditions of drug poisoning.

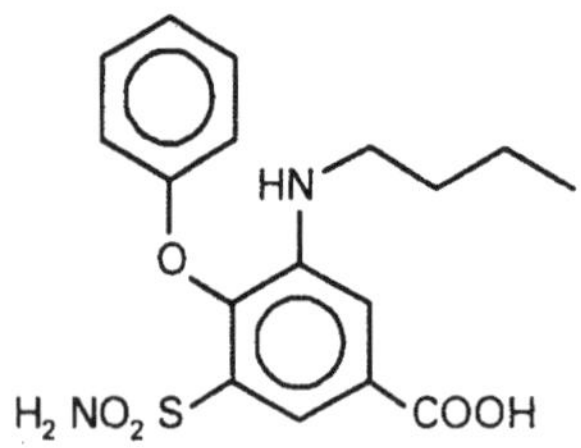

Bumetanide (140)
(Bumex, or Burinex)

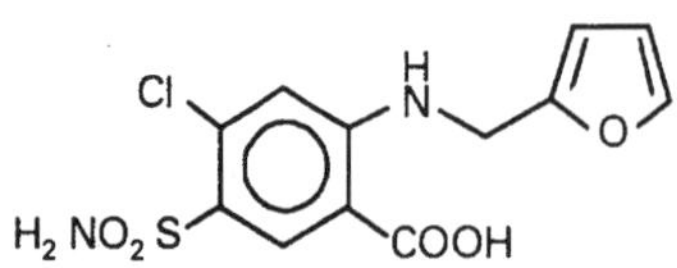

Furosemide (141)
(Lasix)

2.7.5 Carbonic anhydrase inhibitors

The enzyme carbonic anhydrase is present in the kidney, eye and pancreas. Within the proximal tubule cells of the kidney, carbonic anhydrase provides a supply of H^+ ions which are exchanged for sodium in the tubular fluid, so that the body sodium is conserved. The H^+ ions in the tubular fluid then combine with bicarbonate to form carbonic acid (H_2CO_3), which is metabolized to CO_2 and H_2O by carbonic anhydrase. Therefore, the inhibition of carbonic anhydrase reduces the supply of H^+ ions, so that sodium and bicarbonate remain in the tubular fluid.

$$CO_2 + H_2O \xrightleftharpoons{\text{Carbonic anhydrase}} H_2CO_3 \rightleftharpoons H^+ + HCO_3^-$$

This results in alkaline urine with a high sodium bicarbonate content. The increase in sodium excretion leads to diuresis. Further, the increased delivery of sodium to the distal tubule results in an exchange with potassium, causing a loss of potassium. This activity works only for short durations. The continued loss of bicarbonate leads to metabolic acidosis and, therefore, tolerance quickly develops. Metabolic action provides the necessary supply of H^+ ions in the tubular fluid without the action of carbonic anhydrase; at this stage diuresis ceases. Carbonic anhydrase inhibition is, therefore, effective when used intermittently. The following drugs, Acetazolamide (142), Methazolamide (143), Ethoxzolamide (144),and Dichlorphenamide (145) are useful carbonic anhydrase inhibitors.

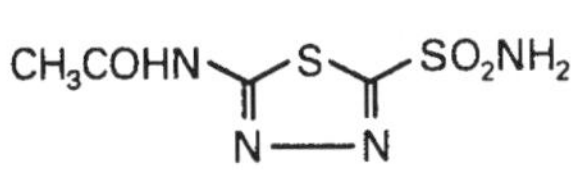

Acetazolamide (142)
(Diomox)

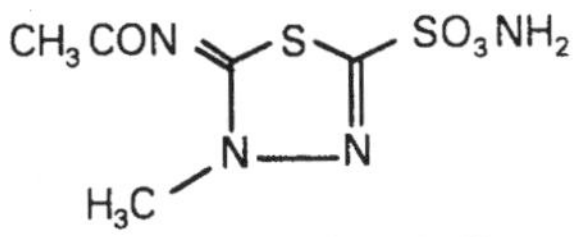

Methazolamide (143)
(Neptazane)

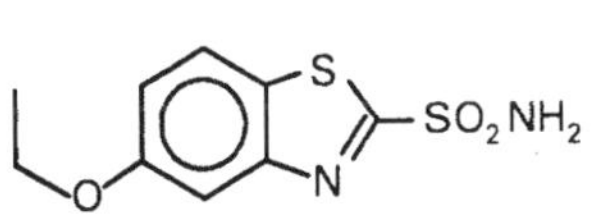

Ethoxzolamide (144)
(Cardrase)

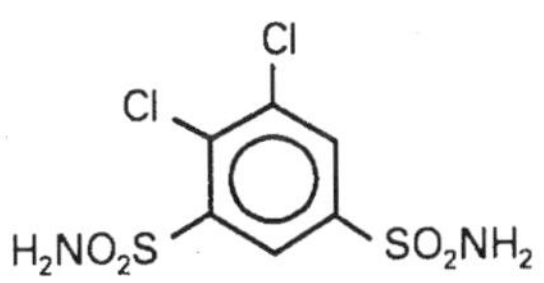

Dichlorphenamide (145)
(Daranide or Oratrol)

2.7.6 Thiazide diuretics

Benzthiadiazines, often called thiazides, are found to possess varying degrees of diuretic action. The main site of action of these compounds is in the distal tubule. The thiazide diuretics inhibit the reabsorption of sodium and chloride ions. For this reason, they are referred to as saluretics (excretion of Na^+ and Cl^- ions). They also inhibit the reabsorption of K^+ and HCO_3^- ions, but to a lesser degree. Thiazide diuretics may induce side effects like hypersensitivity reactions, gastric irritation, nausea, and electrolyte imbalance. Some of the important thiazide diuretics are: Chlorothiazide (146), Benzthiazide (147), Hydrochlorothiazide (148), and Flumethiazide (149).

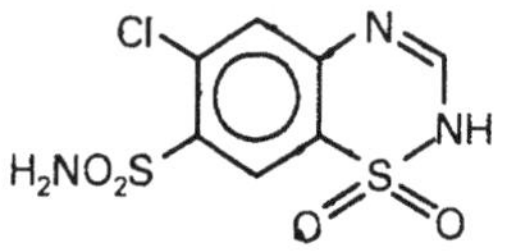

Chlorothiazide (146)
(Diuril)

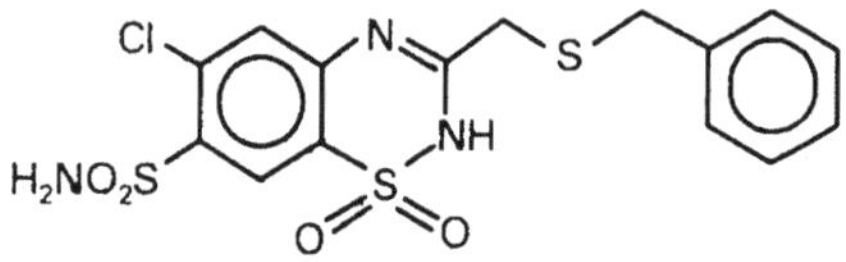

Benzthiazide (147)
(Exna)

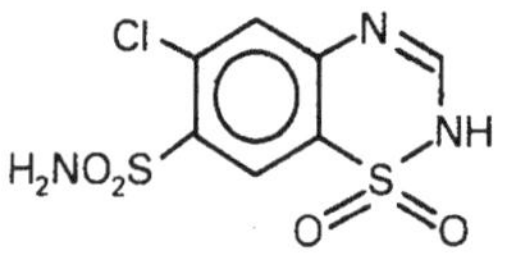

Hydrochlorothiazide (148)
(Esidrix; or Hydro diuril)

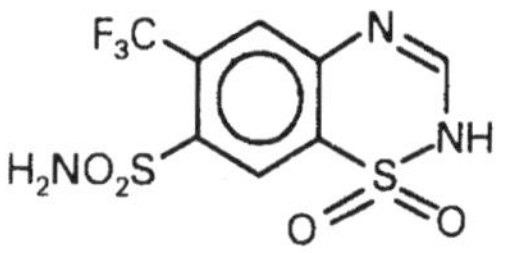

Flumethiazide (149)
(Ademol)

QUESTIONS

I. Main questions

1. Define the terms 'disease' and 'drug'. What, according to the WHO is a drug? What are the requirements of an ideal drug?
2. What are the various sources of drugs? Describe any three in detail.
3. What is a receptor? Describe various types of receptors with examples.
4. What is the structure–activity relationship (SAR) in drugs? Explain in detail, taking Librium as a lead structure.
5. (a) How are CNS drugs classified?
   (b) Explain briefly about analgesics.
6. (a) What is an anaesthetic? What are its ideal characteristics?
   (b) Describe general and local anaesthetics.
7. Explain the role of the autonomic nervous system, giving the classification and suitable examples.
8. (a) Define a diuretic.
   (b) What are the important functions of the kidney?
   (c) What is the role of the nephron in urine formation?

II. Write short notes on

i) Synthetic drugs
ii) Medicinal chemistry
iii) ADME of drugs
iv) Lock and key system of a drug
v) Metabolites
vi) Pharmacophore
vii) Uses of fungi
viii) Gram stain
ix) Antimetabolites

III. Differentiate between

i) Thrombosis and haemorrhage
ii) Depressants and stimulants
iii) Agonist and antagonist
iv) Neurosis and psychosis
v) Prokaryotes and eukaryotes
vi) Bacteria and virus
ix) Metabolite and antimetabolite
viii) Affinity and efficacy

IV. Short answer questions

Briefly describe

i) Psychopharmacological agents
ii) SAR study of sulfa drugs

iii) Pharmacodynamic agents
iv) Hypnotics
v) Non-selective CNS stimulants
vi) Local anaesthetics
vii) General anaesthetics
viii) Analgesics
ix) Antipyretics
x) NSAIDs
xi) Epilepsy
xii) Sedatives
xiii) Parkinson's disease
xiv) Antitussives
xv) Cholinergic drugs
xvi) Antispasmodics
xvii) Sympathetic nervous system
xviii) Hypertension
xix) *Angina pectoris*
xx) Arrythmia
xxi) Cholesterol control
xxii) Anticoagulants
xxiii) Blood clotting mechanism
xxiv) Nephron
xxv) Carbonic anhydrase inhibitors
xxvi) Coagulants
xxvii) Anemia

V. Objective questions

1. State whether the following statements are TRUE or FALSE.
   i. A virus can be seen with the naked eye.
   ii. Some fungi are edible.
   iii. A virus has no cell wall.
   iv. Diuretics are mainly used for increasing the excretion of sodium chloride and water.
   v. Chemically, enzymes are proteins.
   vi. The term 'hypotension' refers to high blood pressure.
   vii. *Angina pectoris* is a heart disease pertaining to the coronary artery.
   viii. Analgesics act by decreasing the threshold of pain.
   ix. Arrythmia means an abnormal heartbeat.
   x. Anticholinergic drugs are also called antispasmodic drugs and are essentially anti-acetylcholine in action.

2. Write the full form of following:
   i) ACE ii) NSAID iii) BP iv) CNS
   v) TB vi) ATP vii) LSD viii) WHO
   ix) DNA

3. Match the following:
   A i. Mycorrhiza (A) Smallpox
   ii. Bacteria (B) Streptomycin

iii. Virus	(C) Mycology
iv. Fungi	(D) Prokaryotes
v. Streptococcus	(E) Biofertilizer
B. i. Louis Pasteur	(A) Pencillin
ii. Gerhard Domagk	(B) Morphine
iii. Paul Ehrlich	(C) Staining procedure
iv. Dioscorides	(D) Smallpox vaccine
v. Alexander Flemming	(E) Receptor
vi. Edward Jenner	(F) ***De Materia Medica***
vii. Christian Gram	(G) Vaccine for rabbies
viii. Surturney	(H) Sulfa drugs
C. i. Blood pressure	(A) Lovastatin
ii. Parkinson's disease	(B) Heparin
iii. Diuretic	(C) Dapsone
iv. Analgesic	(D) Furosemide (Lasix)
v. Bronchodilator	(E) Digoxin
vi. Cardiotonic drug	(F) Livodopa
vii. Cholesterol control	(G) Ibuprofen
viii. Anticoagulant	(H) Captopril
ix. Leprosy	(I) Paracetamol
x. Antipyretic	(J) Salbutamol

VI. Fill in the blanks

1. The degraded products of drugs generated *in vivo* are called __________.
2. The metal ion necessary for blood clotting is ____________.
3. ______________ is the principal chemical neurotransmitter in the parasympathetic division.
4. The instrument used to measure blood pressure is ____________.
5. The enzyme-mediated transformation products of drugs are called ________.
6. In atherosclerosis, ___________ is deposited as fat in the inner linings of the arteries.
7. All red blood cells, white blood cells, and platelets are formed in the ________ __________.
8. The deficiency of iron results in ___________.

9. Those parts of the drug molecule that interact with the receptor are known as ___________.
10. The sudden heritable change of a gene in an organism is known as ___________.
11. Pernicious anaemia is due to the deficiency of ___________.

VII. Choose the correct answer for the following.

1. Haemoglobin present in one of the following cells provides the oxygen-transport mechanism of the blood.
   i. Thrombocytes; ii. Leucocytes; iii. Erythrocytes;
   iv. Platelets ( )
2. The deficiency of which one of the following vitamins increases blood clotting time?
   i. Vitamin A; ii. Vitamin C; iii. Vitamin D; iv. Vitamn K ( )
3. Which of the following drugs is a narcotic analgestic?
   i. Diclofenac; ii. Phenacetin; ii. Paracetamol;
   iv. Morphine ( )
4. Which of the following class of compounds act as a sedative and a hypnotic?
   i. Benzodiazepines; ii. Antibiotics; iii. Coumarins;
   iv. Steroids ( )
5. The drugs used to control the excessive quantity of acetylcholine are called
   i. Cholinergic drugs; ii. Psychotomimetics; iii. Antispasmodics;
   iv. Analeptics ( )
6. The range of serum cholesterol in normal individual is
   i. 190–250 mg/dL; ii. 120–80 mm; iii. 100–150 mm;
   iv. 145–90 mm ( )
7. Phylloquinone is a
   i. Xanthine diuretic; ii. Anasthetic; iii. Sedative;
   iv. Vitamin K ( )
8. In blood clotting, the actual chemical which coagulates the blood is
   i. Heparin; ii. Coumarin; iii. Fibrin; iv. Prothrombin ( )
9. The enzyme carbonic anhydrase catalyzes the generation of
   i. HCl; ii. H_2CO_3; iii. H_2sO_4; iv. CH_3COOH ( )
10. The approximate number of nephrons present in each kidney is
    i. one million; ii. one thousand; iii. one hundred;
    iv. two ( )

Answers to objective questions

V.1. i-F; ii-T; iii-T; iv-T; v-T; vi-F; vii-T; viii-F; ix-T; x-T
F = False; T = True

2. i. Angiotensin Converting Enzyme
   ii. Non-steroidal Anti-inflammatory Drugs
   iii. Blood Pressure
   iv. Central Nervous System
   v. Tuberculosis Bacillus
   vi. Adonisine Triphosphate
   vii. Lysergic Acid Diethylamide
   viii. World Health Organization
   ix. Deoxyribonucleic acid

3. A. i-E; ii-D; iii-A; iv-C; v-B
   B. i-G; ii-H; iii-E; iv-F; v-A; vi-D; vii-C; viii-B
   C. i-H; ii-F; iii-D; iv-G; v-j; vi-E; vii-A; viii-B; ix-C; x-I

VI. 1. Metabolites; 2. Ca^{2+}; 3. Acetylcholine;
4. Sphygmomanometer; 5. Metabolites; 6. Cholesterol;
7. Bone marrow; 8. Anemia; 9. Pharmacophore;
10. Mutation; 11. Vitamin B_{12}

VII. 1-iii; 2-iv; 3-iv; 4-i; 5-iii; 6-i; 7-iv; 8-iii; 9-ii; 10-i

3 VITAMINS, HORMONES AND SYNTHETIC DRUGS

3.1 Introduction

The average life expectancy of human beings has been on the rise. One of the major reasons for this is the widespread use of drugs. Over the past hundred years, the most remarkable application is the increasing use of organic compounds as drugs. The term **chemotherapy** (shorter version of chemical therapy) is generally used for the treatment of diseases by chemicals, caused due to microbial infections (see page 42). Drugs are broadly classified into three groups:

i) Chemotherapeutic drugs; ii) Pharmacodynamic agents; iii) Vitamins and hormones

In this chapter, a brief account of vitamins and hormones is given. The synthesis of some of the common drugs and their therapeutic uses are presented. Penicillin, as an example of a natural drug, is also described.

The synthesis and mechanism of action of two chemotherapeutic drugs of the class of antibacterials are described in this chapter.

3.2 Vitamins: a class of nutrients

Nutrients

The human body is considered as a **live chemical laboratory** in which several biochemical processes take place at any given time. For proper biochemical processes, we need a balanced diet that includes carbohydrates, proteins, fats, minerals and water. These are different classes of nutrients that are necessary for good health.

Carbohydrates provide energy for the body (approximately 4 KCal of energy is produced by the oxidation of 1 gm of glucose). **Proteins** are essential for building up the structural units of the body, called cells. Enzymes, some hormones, antibodies, transport molecules (such as as hemoglobin) and fibrinogen (for blood clotting) are all protein molecules. **Fats** serve as 'reservoirs' of food. Fatty cells are specialized ones that store food, mostly in the form of triglycerides. **Minerals** are nutrient elements such as calcium, phosphorus, magnesium, iron, iodine, etc. They are the constituents of enzymes, co-enzymes, transport molecules, etc. **Water** is the medium for most of the biochemical reactions in the body, the transport of nutrients and waste products. In addition to carbohydrates, proteins, fats, minerals and water, it has been ascertained that the body requires certain other nutritional factors called **vitamins**.

Vitamins

The term 'vitamine' is derived from the word *vital* (meaning life) and *amine*. As the first discovered members of this class of compounds contain amino groups, these were named vitamines. Later, it was found that all of them do not have amino groups. Hence, the letter 'e' was deleted from vitamine. Now, it is spelled *as vitamin*. ***Vitamins*** are a class of nutrients / dietary factors that can not be biosynthesized by the human body (except D_2) and are supplied through our diet. These are essential for the normal functioning of the body, and are produced by plants. Some of the vitamins are synthesized while others are extracted from microorganisms.

The human body needs vitamins in balanced proportions and in small quantities. The deficiency of a particular vitamin causes a specific disease(s) (Table 3.1). The treatment of deficiency diseases by supplementing the diet with the necessary vitamins is known as **vitamin therapy**. Therefore, vitamins can be considered as drugs if they fall short in the body; otherwise, they are nutrients.

On the other hand, an excess consumption of vitamins may cause side effects (**hyper-vitaminosis**). For example, an excess of vitamin A causes irritability and dry skin. An overdose of vitamin D can cause pain in the bones. Extra amounts of fat-soluble vitamins are stored in the fatty tissues, especially in the liver; water-soluble vitamins tend to be excreted.

3.2.1 Classification of vitamins

On the basis of solubility in fat or water, vitamins are broadly divided into **fat-soluble vitamins** (lipophilic) and **water-soluble vitamins** (hydrophilic), respectively. Vitamins A, D, E and K are fat-soluble; whereas vitamins B-complex and C, are water-soluble. The structure of the former class of vitamins consists of a higher portion of hydrocarbon and less polar group(s), thus making them fat-soluble. The latter group of vitamins have a larger number of polar groups and, hence, are soluble in water (fats are less polar than water).

3.2.2 Structure, biochemical functions, deficiency diseases and sources of vitamins

The structures of various vitamins have been established. Vitamin D_2 is produced in the skin from ergosterol (a steroid) on exposure to sunlight. For this reason, vitamin D is some times called the *sunshine vitamin* (Fig. 3.1). (There is a misconception that vitamin D is present in sunlight !).The

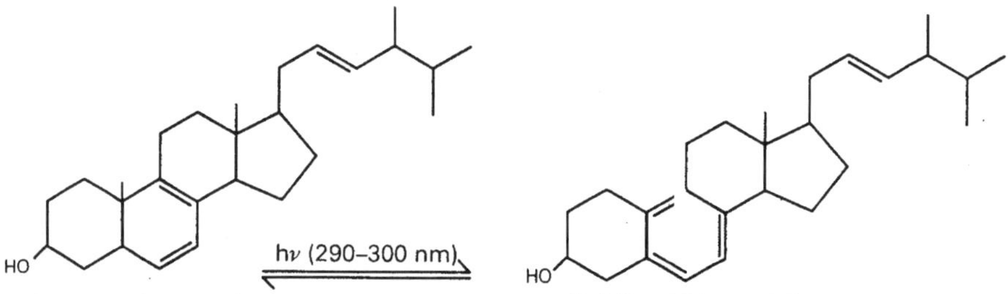

Ergosterol (a steroid) Calciferol (Ergocalciferol) (Vitamin D_2)

Fig. 3.1 *Isomerization of Ergosterol to Vitamin D_2 in the presence of light.*

structures of some of the vitamins along with their biochemical functions, diseases caused due to deficiency, and sources are presented in Table 3.1.

Table 3.1 *Names, Structures, Biochemical Functions, Deficiency Symptoms and Sources of some Vitamins*

Names and Structures of Vitamins	– **Biochemical Functions** – **Deficiency Effects** – **Sources**
	A. Fat-soluble Vitamins
Retinol (Vitamin A) 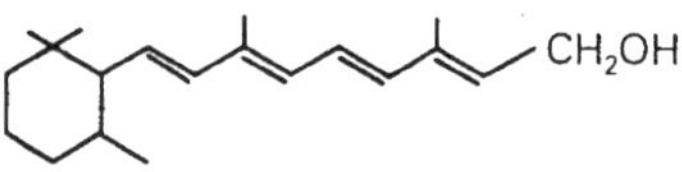 	– Prevents night blindness by regeneration of rhodopsin (visual purple) and protects the eye from infection – Deficiency causes light sensitivity, night blindness, xerophthalmia – Fish, liver, eggs, butter, cheese; β-carotene in carrots is a provitamin (vitamin precursor)
Calciferol (Vitamin D_2) 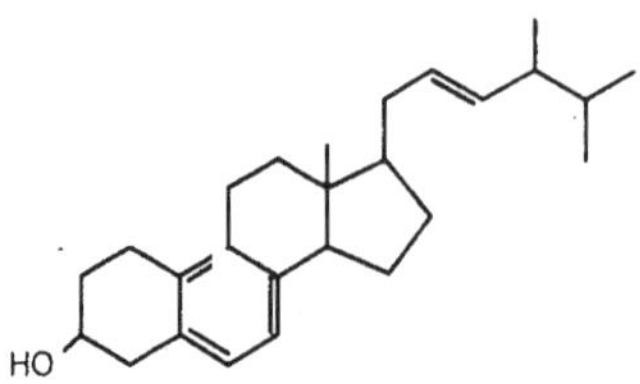 	– Aids in Ca and P metabolism and is essential in building strong bones – Deficiency causes rickets – Cod liver oil, irradiated ergosterol (vitamin D_2) as a milk supplement

α-Tocopherol (Vitamin E)

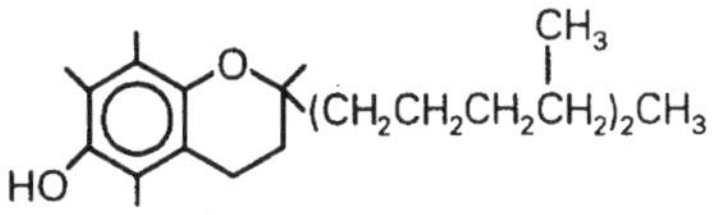

- Antioxidant (prevents oxidation, e.g., of fats), maintains RBC membranes
- Oedema and anemia in infants; sterility (Vitamin E is often called the *antisterility vitamin*, as it is responsible for normal reproductive function)
- Wheatgerm oil, green vegetables, egg-yolk, meat, nuts

Phylloquinone (Vitamin K_1)

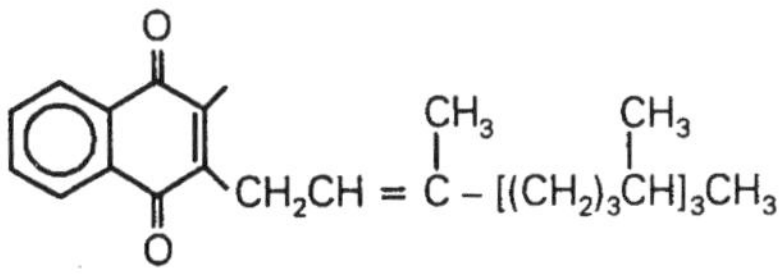

- Aids in synthesis of prothrombin (blood coagulant) Slows clotting of blood and hemorrhage
- Cauliflower, leafy vegetables

B. Water-soluble vitamins

B-Complex

Thiamine (Vitamin B_1)

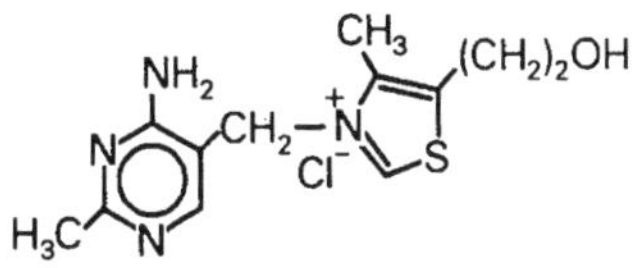

- Carbohydrate metabolism, proper functioning of heart and circulatory system
- Deficiency causes beriberi (i.e., polyneuritis, resulting in muscle paralysis; enlargement of the heart, and finally heart failure)
- Cereal grains, legumes, milk, nuts

Niacin (Vitamin B_3)

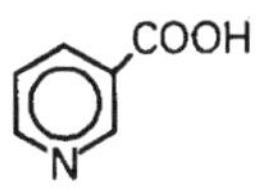

Nicotinic acid

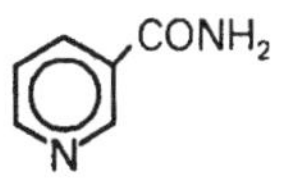

Nicotinamide

- Metabolism of carbohydrates, fats and proteins
- Deficiency causes pellagra (symptoms are diarrhea, dermatitis and dementia (loss of memory)
- Yeast, liver, peanuts, soyabeans, potatoes

Pantothenic acid (Vitamin B_5)

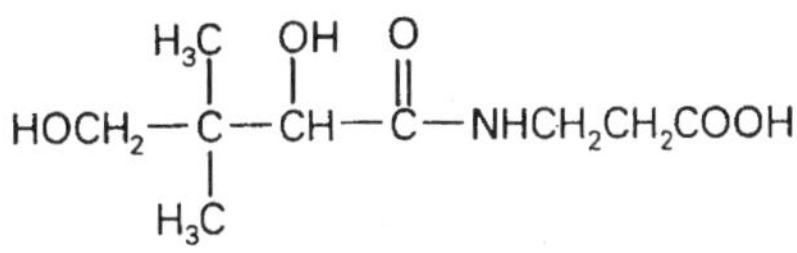

- Useful in the synthesis of sex hormones, heme, cholesterol, fatty acids, amino acids
- Causes retarted growth, gastrointestinal disturbances, (possibly) emotional problems
- Yeast, mushrooms, egg-yolk, nuts, liver

Vitamin B_6

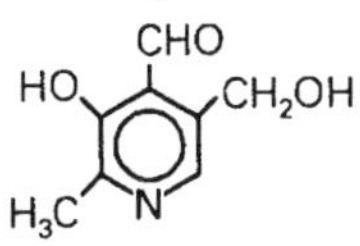

Pyridoxal

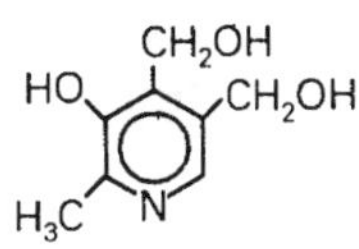

Pyridoxol

- Necessary for growth and healthy nervous system
- Causes dermatitis, irritability and increased susceptibility to infections, weakness
- Egg, liver, yeast, peas, beans, milk

Folic acid (Vitamin B_9) 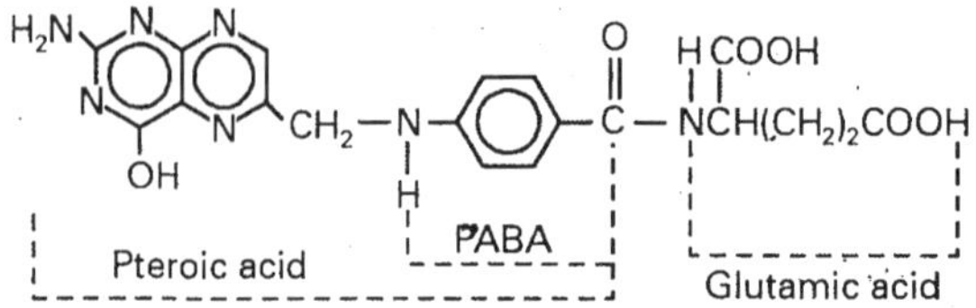	– Coenzyme related to growth, important in proper development of RBC – Causes anemias (treatment of megaloblastic anemia, characterized by RBC) – Liver, kidney, mushrooms, yeast, green leafy vegetables
Ascorbic acid (Vitamin C) 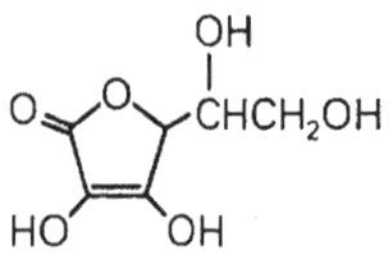	– Act as a reducing agent, complexes with metal ions, resists disease, helps in healing wounds – Causes scurvy (symptoms are swollen legs, red-spotted skin, rotten gums, black lungs and damaged liver) – Citrus fruits, tomatoes, green pepper

*see Appendix for Vitamin B_{12} (cobalamine)

3.3 *Hormones: the chemical messengers*

The term *hormone* is derived from the Greek word *hormaein* (which means 'to set in motion'). Hormones are chemical messengers secreted in small quantities (nanograms to milligrams per day) by ductless glands called the **endocrine glands** of the body. Unlike vitamins, hormones are produced in the human body. The pituitary, parathyroid, thyroid, adrenal, pancreas are some of the endocrine glands present in humans. Hormones perform varied physiological functions: increase or decrease the rate of reaction, control growth, metabolism and reproduction, and many other functions of the body (Table 3.2).

Structurally, all hormones are not alike; they have diverse structures just like vitamins (Fig. 3.2). They may be classified according to structure:

i) amino acid (L-tyrosine) based hormones, e.g., thyroxin
ii) polypeptide and protein-based hormones, e.g., insulin
iii) steroidal hormones, e.g., testosterone

Any deficiency of a hormone causes a disease. *Hormone therapy* (supplementing hormones as drugs) is used to treat such diseases. The physiological functions and the glands that secrete the hormones are represented in Table 3.2.

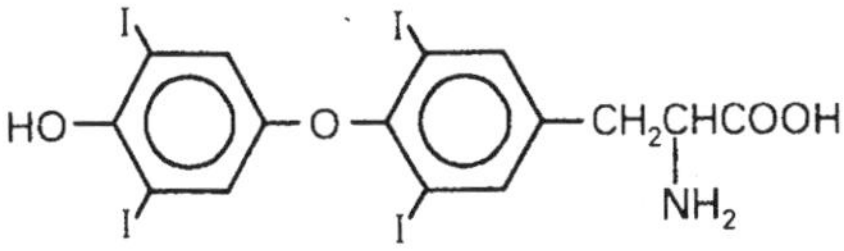

Thyroxine
(an amino acid derivative)

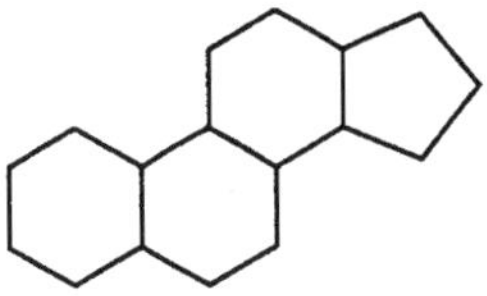

skeletal structure of a steriod

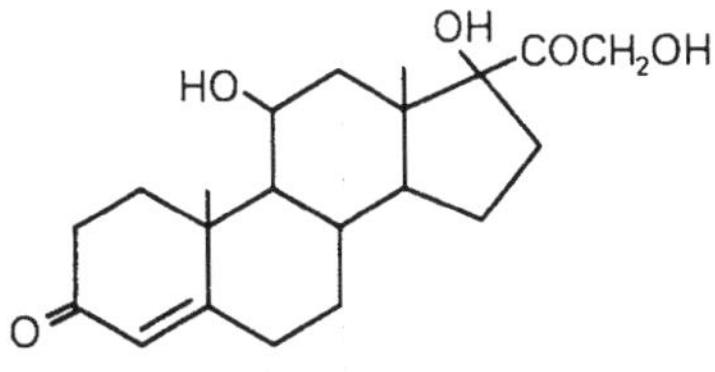

Cortisol (a steroidal hormone secreted by the cortex of the adrenal glands)

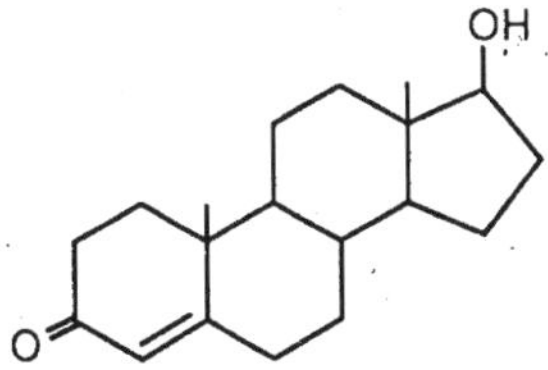

Testosterone (a male sex hormone)

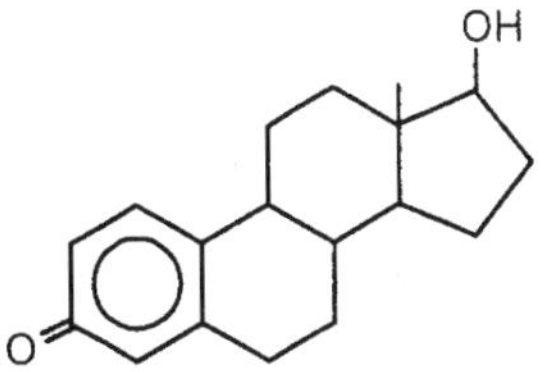

Estradiol (a female sex hormone)

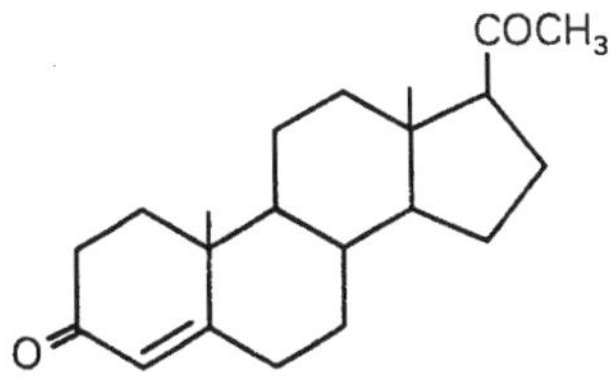

Progesterone (a female sex hormone)

Fig. 3.2 *Structures of some hormones.*

Table 3.2 *A few Hormones, Glands that Secrete them, and their Physiological Effects*

Name of the Hormone	Glands (Tissues)	Physiological Effects (Diseases)
Thyroxine (amino acid based)	Thyroid*	Regulates the rate of oxygen consumption and cellular metabolism (goitre)
Oxytocin (polypeptide-based)	Pituitary (posterior lobe)	Stimulates secretion of milk and contraction of smooth muscles of the uterus
Insulin (polypeptide-based)	Pancreas (beta cells)	Increases cell usage of glucose, glycogen storage (diabetes)
Cortisol (steroidal hormone)	Adrenal gland (cortex)	Stimulates conversion of proteins into carbohydrates
Testosterone (steroidal hormone)	Testes	Stimulates and maintains male sex characteristics

(continues...)

Table 3.2 *(...contd.)*

Estradiol (steroidal hormone)	Ovaries (follicles)	Stimulates female sex characteristics and regulates the menstrual cycle
Progesterone (steroidal hormone)	Ovaries (corpus luteum)	Regulates the menstrual cycle and maintains pregnancy

*Inadequate thyroid secretion causes **hypothyroidism** which, in turn, causes cretinism, characterized by the retardation of mental, physical and sexual development in infants. On the other hand, excessive secretion of thyroid results in **hyperthyroidism**. Iodine is essential to produce thyroxine and a deficiency of iodine causes the enlargement of thyroid. This abnormality is called **goitre**. To overcome this problem, iodized salt can be used which consists of approximately 0.1% NaI or KI.

3.4 *Synthetic and natural drugs*

Drugs are not only obtained from natural sources, i.e., plants and animals (**natural drugs**), but also synthesized in a chemical laboratory (**synthetic drugs**). Natural drugs that are partly structurally modified are called **semisynthetic drugs**. There are approximately 2000 compounds that are in use worldwide as drugs. Most of them are synthetic drugs, of which **achiral drugs** are more than **chiral drugs**. Among chiral drugs, the majority are used as **racemates** and a few are used as single **enantiomers**. In contrast to synthetic drugs, natural and semisynthetic drugs are chiral and single enantiomers.

3.5 *Synthetic drugs*

The foregoing discussion involves laboratory synthesis and therapeutic activity of the following drugs:

1) Sulphanilamide
2) Paracetamol
3) Aspirin
4) Oil of Wintergreen
5) Mephensin
6) Ibuprofen
7) L-DOPA
8) Albuterol
9) Analgin
10) Metachloropromide
11) Chloroquine
12) Chloropromazine
13) Phenobarbital
14) Omeprazole
15) Nifedipine
16) Ciprofloxacin

A synthetic plan is also provided, for most of the drugs listed here, for a better understanding of the syntheses.

3.5.1 Sulphanilamide: an example of a sulpha drug

Sulphonamides that are useful as drugs are called **sulpha drugs**. Sulphonamides are amides of sulphonic acid. The general structural formula of a sulpha drug is shown on the following page.

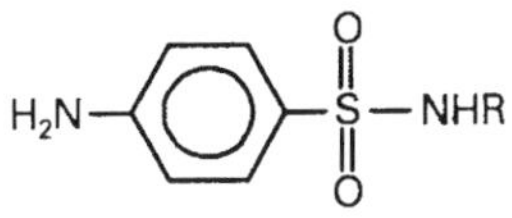

Sulphanilamide (R = H) is 4-aminobenzenesulphonamide. Its structure and synthetic plan is provided in Fig. 3.3.

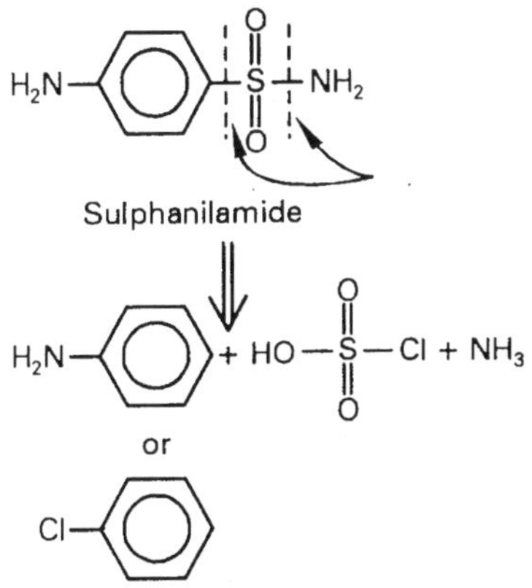

Fig. 3.3 *Structure and synthetic plan of sulphanilamide.*

A large number of sulphonamides have been synthesized and tested; a few of them are used as drugs. One such drugs is sulphanilamide. Other sulpha drugs include sulphathiazole (R = 2-thiozolyl), sulphapyridine (R = 2-pyridyl), sulphadiazine (R = 2-diazinyl). These drugs with heterocyclic substituted rings are more active than simple sulphanilamide (see page 47). Sulpha drugs were extensively used as anti-bacterials between 1940–1960.

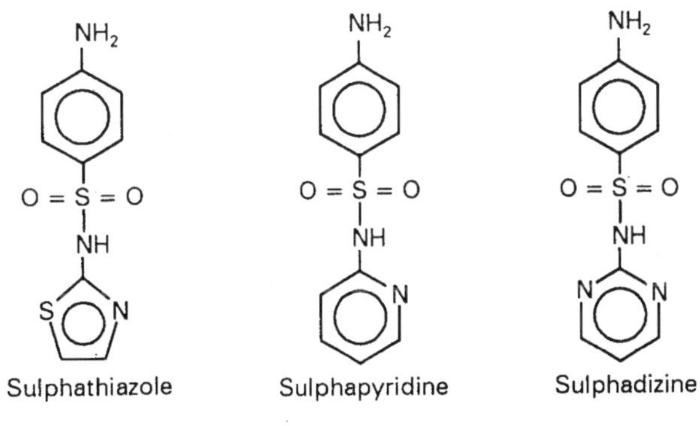

Synthesis From the synthetic plan (Fig. 3.3), it is evident that sulphanilamide synthesis can be achieved in two different ways—from aniline and chlorobenzene.

Method A (from aniline; Scheme 3.1a) The acetylation of aniline gives acetanilide which, on chlorosulphonation, yields 4-methylcarboxamido-1-benzenesulphonyl chloride. This drug intermediate is subjected to ammonolysis and deacetylation (through hydrolysis) to give sulphanilamide.

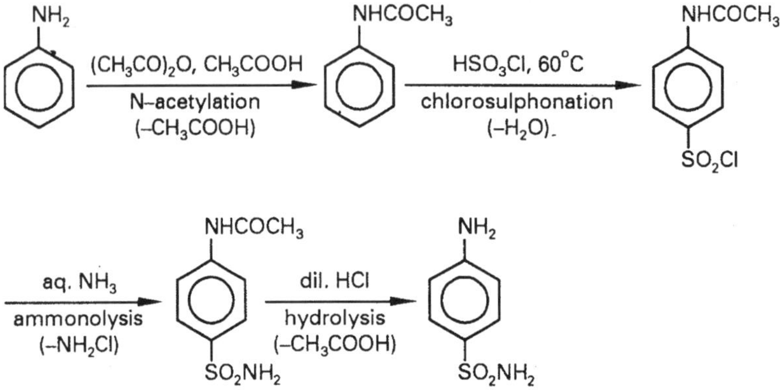

Scheme 3.1a Synthesis of sulphanilamide.

Method B (from chlorobenzene; Scheme 3.1b) Alternatively, sulphanilamide can also be synthesized from chlorobenzene in two steps. In the first step, chlorosulphonation of chlorobenzene gives 4-chlorobenzenesulphonyl chloride. This intermediate, in the second step, is subjected to ammonolysis (reaction with ammonia) to yield sulphanilamide.

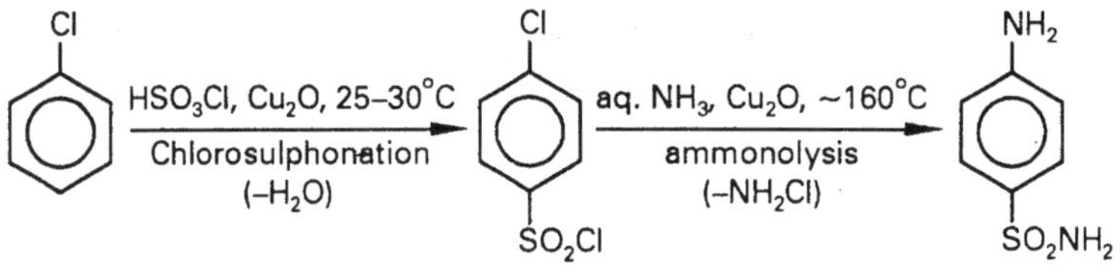

Scheme 3.1b Synthesis of sulphanilamide.

Therapeutic activity Sulphanilamide is a *bactereostatic drug,* i.e., one which inhibits the growth of bacteria. The mechanism of the drug action is briefly described here. Bacteria synthesize *folic acid* (vitamin B_9) which is necessary for their growth. The key compound for the synthesis of folic acid is p-aminobenzoic acid (PABA). The drug, sulphanilamide, is a structural analog of PABA. Bacteria can not discriminate between the two and, hence, uses sulphanilamide instead of PABA (an example of mistaken identity!). As a result, pseudo-folic acid (wrong folic acid) is synthesized, inhibiting further growth of bacteria. The structure – activity relationships of these class of compounds has been described earlier (page 47).

3.5.2 Paracetamol (Acetaminophen): antipyretic and analgesic

Paracetamol is N-(4-hydroxyphenyl)-ethanamide (4-hydroxyacetanilide). The synthetic methods involve starting from phenol or 1-chloro-4-nitrobenzene, as shown in the synthetic plan (Fig. 3.4).

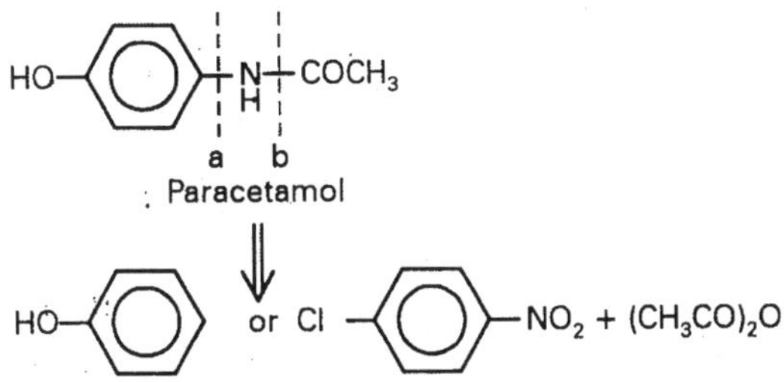

Fig. 3.4 *The structure and synthetic plan of paracetamol.*

Synthesis

Method A (from phenol; Scheme 3.2a) Nitrosation of phenol gives 4-nitrosophenol which, on reduction, yields 4-aminophenol as a drug intermediate. This compound, on selective acetylation (acetylation of the amino group but not the hydroxy group), results in paracetamol.

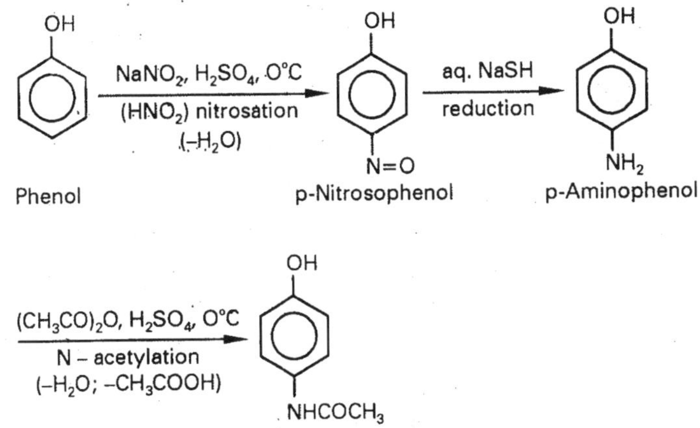

Scheme 3.2a Synthesis of paracetamol starting from phenol.

Method B (from 1-chloro-4-nitrobenzene; Scheme 3.2b) The first step involves treatment of 1-chloro-4-nitrobenzene with aq.NaOH to yield 4-nitrophenol. This reaction is an example of aromatic nucleophilic substitution (S_NAr). In the second step, the nitro group of 4-nitrophenol is reduced to an amino group using H_2 in the presence of Pd-C as a catalyst, and the amino group is converted to acetamido group in presence of acetic anhydride. Both reduction and acetylation take place in one step.

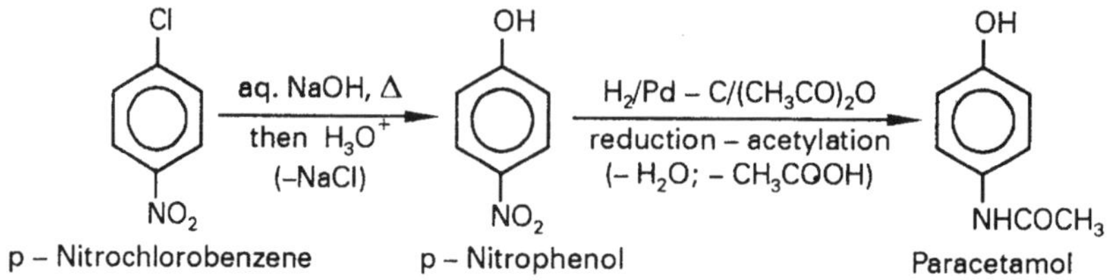

Scheme 3.2b Synthesis of paracetamol starting from p-nitrochlorobenzene.

Therapeutic activity Paracetamol is both an analgesic (pain-killing) and an antipyretic (fever- reducing) agent. It acts on the hypothalamus to reduce temperature—heat dissipation increases as a result of vasodilation and increased peripherial blood flow.

3.5.3 Aspirin (Acetylsalicylic acid): the first synthetic drug; synthesized in 1853 and introduced as a drug in 1899

The bark of the tree *Salis alba ulgaris* (willow) has been used from time immemorial to reduce fever. It contains "salicin" which is the glycoside of salicylic acid.

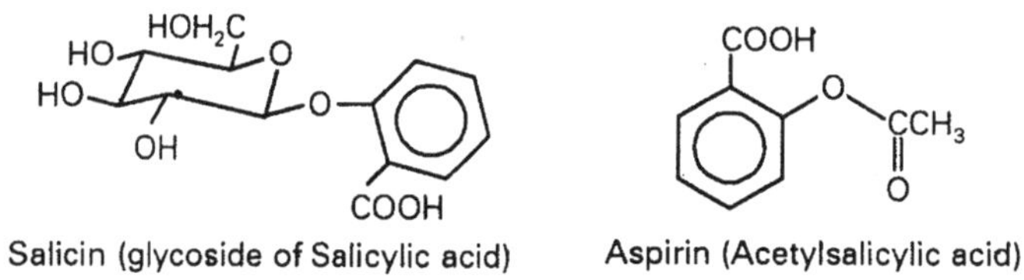

In the body, salicin is hydrolyzed into salicyclic acid, which is responsible for its antipyretic and analgesic activity. The Bayer company synthesized several derivatives of salicylic acid and found that acetylsalicyclic acid (Aspirin) has good antipyretic, analgesic activity and also anti-inflammatory activity.

Synthesis Aspirin is synthesized by acid-catalyzed acetylation of salicyclic acid, using acetic anhydride (Scheme 3.3). (Salicylic acid is, itself, synthesized from phenol using the Kolbe-Schmidt reaction.)

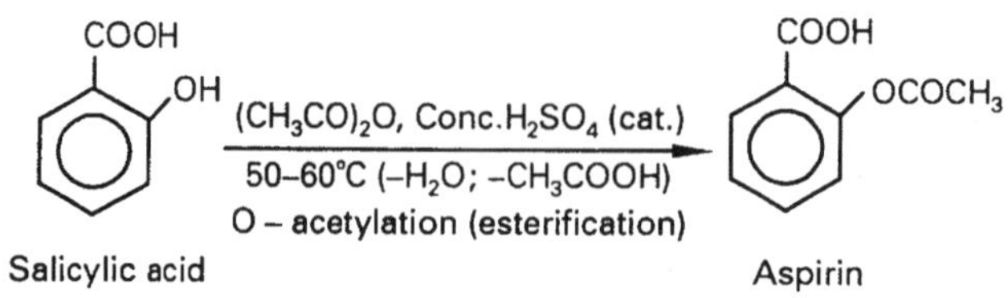

Scheme 3.3 Synthesis of aspirin.

Therapeutic activity Aspirin is both analgesic and antipyretic (it falls at the mild end of the spectrum of analgesic activity). It is probably one the most widely used drugs in the world for pain relief.

Aspirin, in the gastrointestinal tract, is hydrolyzed into salicylic acid and absorbed into the bloodstream. Salicylic acid is a metabolite of aspirin, and inhibits the enzymatic activity of *prostaglandin synthase*. This results in the controlled production of prostaglandins, which are responsible for the sensation of pain. The result is that the impulses responsible for pain are suppressed. Salicylic acid cannot be used as a drug directly. It is sour and causes severe intestinal bleeding, when taken orally; Aspirin does not cause such bleeding. This is the advantage of aspirin over salicyclic acid as a drug; Aspirin is a prodrug.

3.5.4 Oil of wintergreen: ointment for lumbago, sciatica and rheumatism

Oil of wintergreen is the common name of a plant as well as one of its constituents, methyl salicylate.

Synthesis Oil of wintergreen is synthesized by the esterification of salicylic acid using methanol which is catalyzed by conc.H_2SO_4 (Scheme 3.4).

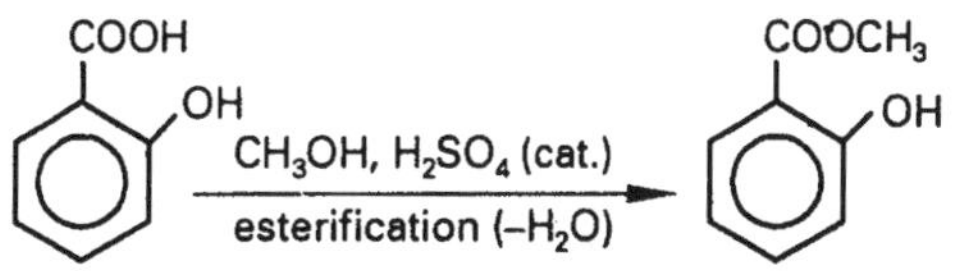

Salicylic acid Methylsalicylate

Scheme 3.4 Synthesis of methylsalicylate.

Therapeutic uses Oil of wintergreen is used in the form of ointments for pain relief in lumbago, sciatica and rheumatism. It is readily absorbed through the skin.

3.5.5 Mephensin: a muscle relaxant

Mephensin is 3-(2-methylphenoxy)-1,2-propanediol (also known as 3-(o-tolyloxy)- propane-1, 2-diol). The structure and synthetic plan of mephensin are shown in Fig 3.5.

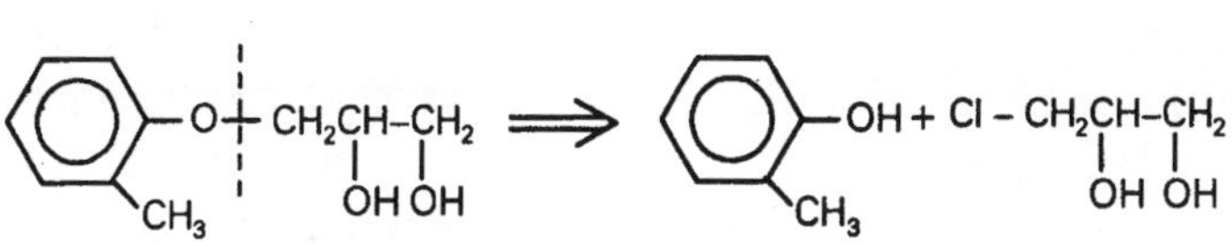

Mephensin

Fig. 3.5 *Synthetic plan for mephensin.*

Synthesis Mephensin is synthesized from o-cresol. o-Cresol is treated with aq.NaOH to convert into sodium salt, which undergoes nucleophilic substitution with 3-chloro-1,2-propanediol, to give mephensin (Williamson Synthesis) (Scheme 3.5).

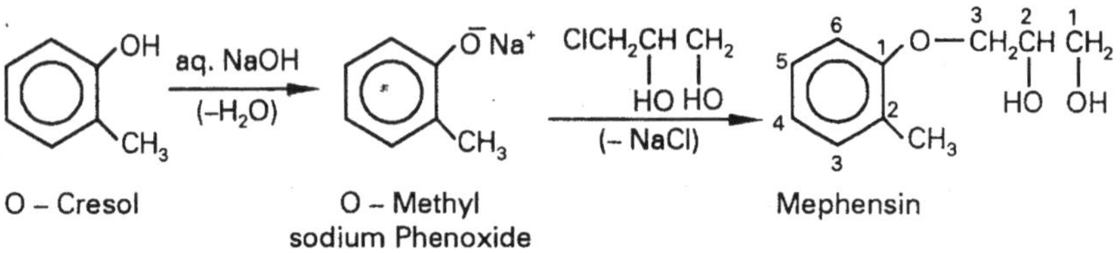

Scheme 3.5 Synthesis of mephensin.

Therapeutic activity It is a potent muscle relaxant.

3.5.6 Ibuprofen: an anti-inflammatory drug, available in pure enantiomeric and racemic form

Ibuprofen is 2-(4-isobutylphenyl)-propanoic acid. It consists of one chiral carbon and exists in two enantiomeric forms (R and S). The structure of Ibuprofen (R and S enantiomers) and its synthetic plan is given in Fig. 3.6.

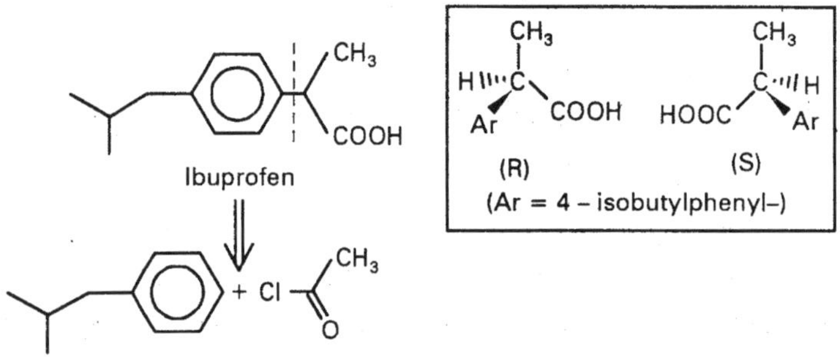

Fig. 3.6 *Structure and synthetic plan of ibuprofen.*

Synthesis Ibuprofen is synthesized from isobutylbenzene, first by Friedel-Crafts acetylation of 4-isobutylbenzene to yield 1-(4-isobutylphenyl)-1-ethanone. This intermediate is converted into Ibuprofen by two possible synthetic routes (Route 1 or 2) (Scheme 3.6).

Route 1 involves the formation of cyanohydrin which, on reduction followed by hydrolysis, gives ibuprofen. *Route 2* involves reduction of the acetophenone derivative to the corresponding alcohol which, on reaction with PX_3(X = Cl or Br), gives the corresponding halocompound. This compound, when subjected to reaction with NaCN and then hydrolysis, gives ibuprofen.

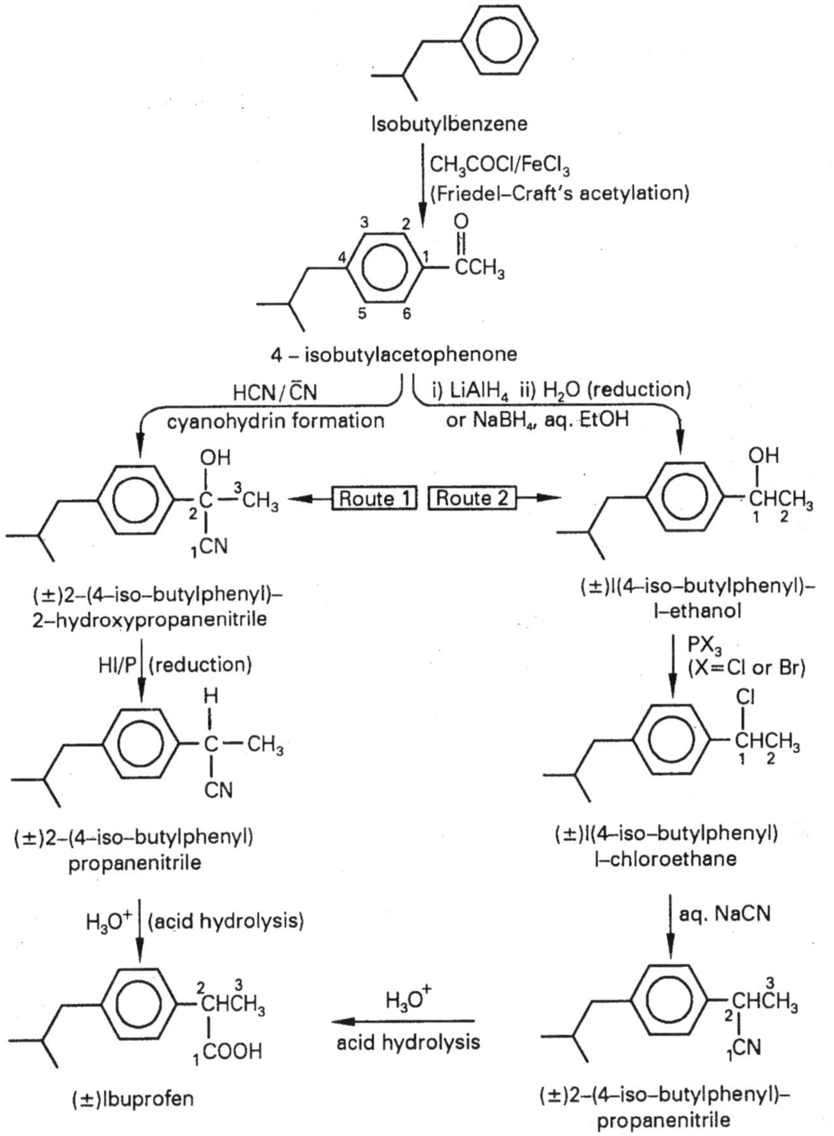

Scheme 3.6 Synthesis of ibuprofen.

Therapeutic activity Ibuprofen is a **n**on-steroidal **a**nti-**i**nflammatory drug (NSAID). In terms of pharmocology, ibuprofen inhibits platelet aggregation and prolongs bleeding time. The drug activity is due to S(+) enantiomer, whereas R(-) enantiomer is inactive and also non-toxic. Ibuprofen is marketed in the S(+) form as well as its racemic form, which is cheaper than the S(+) form. Ibuprofen also shows **analgesic** activity (general pain reliever).

Drugs that show similar theraupetic properties to ibuprofen have been synthesized. Two of them are ketoprofen and naproxen.

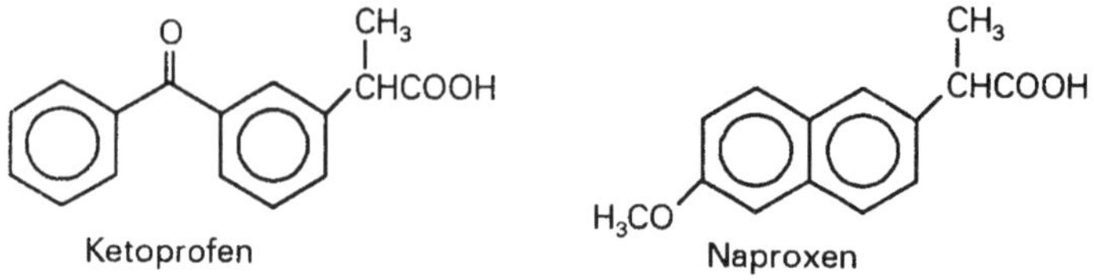

3.5.7 L-dopa - cures Parkinson's disease; L(or S)-dopa is active whereas D(or R)- dopa is toxic

L-Dopa (**D**ihydr**o**xy**p**henyl **a**lanine) is systematically known as (L)3-(3, 4-dihydroxy-phenyl)-2-aminopropanoic acid. Structurally, it resembles the naturally occuring amino acids, L-tyrosine and L-phenylalanine. The Fischer-projection formulae of these three compounds are represented below.

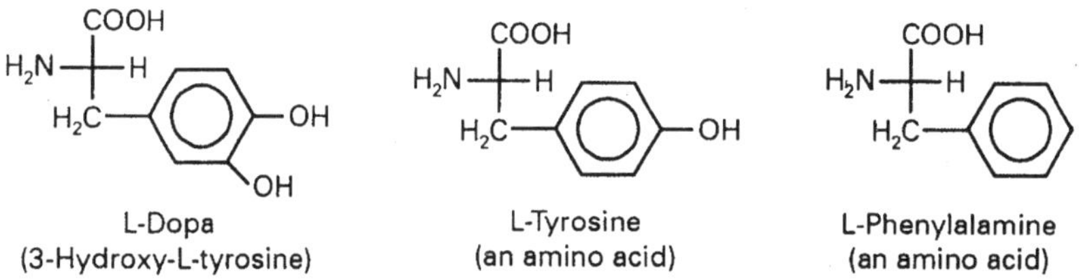

L-dopa has one chiral carbon. In terms of absolute configuration, it is called (S)-3 (3,4-dihydroxyphenyl)-2-aminopropanoic acid (S-dopa). Since (S)-dopa is levorotatory, it is also referred to as (S)(-)-dopa (Fig. 3.7 gives its synthetic plan).

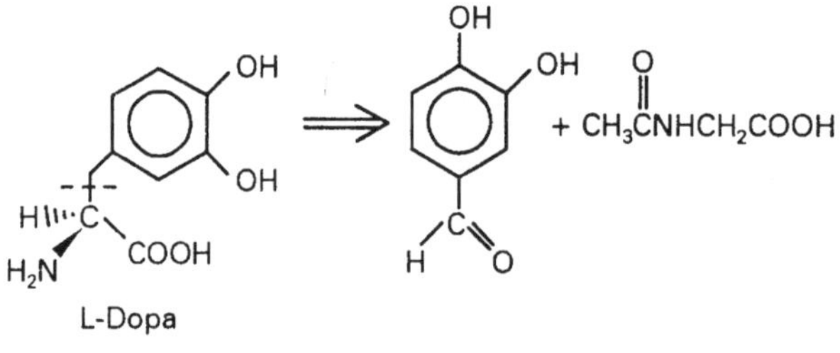

Fig. 3.7 *Synthetic plan for L-Dopa.*

Synthesis L-dopa is synthesized from 3, 4-dihydroxybenzaldehyde and N-acetyl glycine by the Perkin type of condensation, followed by saponification (basic hydrolysis of an ester group). Dehydration of the intermediate yields a mixture of geometric isomers (E/Z isomers). Hydrogenation of the mixture, using H_2/Pd-C (catalyst), gives the racemic

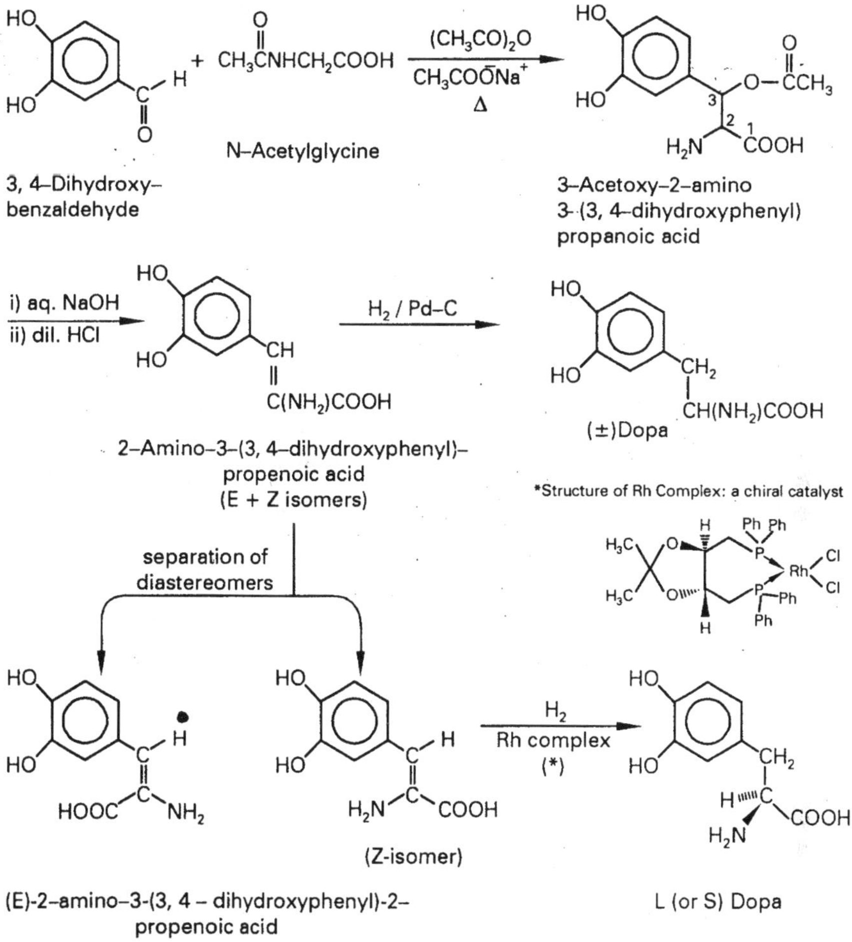

Scheme 3.7 Synthesis of L-Dopa.

dopa. Hydrogenation of the Z-isomer, obtained in the pure state after separation, using a chiral catalyst (a Rhodium complex), gives (S)-dopa (L-Dopa) selectively (Scheme 3.7). This is an example of asymmetric synthesis (the synthesis of an optically active product from achiral starting material using an optically active reagent and/or catalyst, is known as asymmetric synthesis).

Therapeutic activity L-dopa cures Parkinson's disease (see box) caused by the deficiency of dopamine, which is one of the neurotransmitters in the brain.

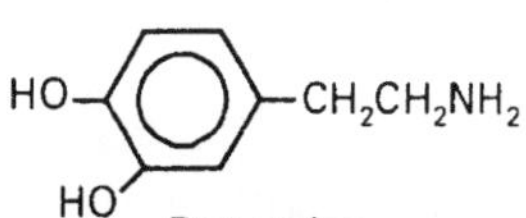

Dopamine

Levo dopa (or L-dopa) penetrates the Central Nervous System(CNS) and is enzymatically converted into dopamine in the basal ganglia. Dopamine itself cannot be directly used as a drug, because it cannot penetrate into the CNS from the bloodstream. L-dopa enters into the cerebral fluid where it is decarboxylated to dopamine through the action of an enzyme. (D)(+)-dopa does not have any therapeutic activity; moreover, it is toxic. For this reason, S-dopa (L-dopa) alone is used as a drug, but not in its racemic form. This is an example where one of the enantiomers is useful as a drug and the other enantiomer is not.

Parkinson's disease

First described as a 'shaking palsy' in 1871 by James Parkinson (hence the name, Parkinson's disease), this disease is a neurological disorder associated with two areas of the brain: (1) *Substantia* nigra (situated at the centre of the brain); (2) *Striatum* (situated near the base of the skull). Parkinsonism is characterized by a loss of the pigmented cells of the *substantia nigra,* with an associated decrease in the concentration of dopamine. The striatium is also rich in acetylcholine—a neurohormone. For the normal functioning of the brain there should be a balance

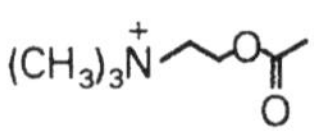

Acetylcholine

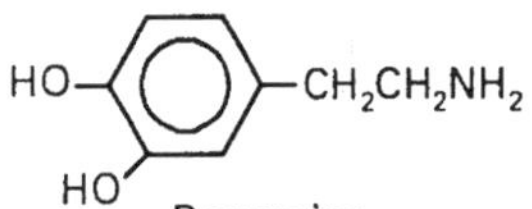

Dopamine

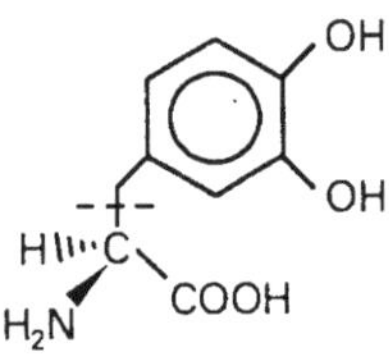

L - Dopa

between the actions of dopamine and acetylcholine. If there is a deficiency of dopamine, this balance would be affected. This causes the primary symptoms of the disease, i.e., tremors, stiffness, slowness of moment, and difficulty in walking. At the advanced stage, the secondary symptoms are depression, senility, postural deformity and loss of speech.

3.5.8 Albuterol (Salbutamol): a bronchodilator

Albuterol is 2-(*tert*-butylamino)-1-(4-hydroxy-3-hydroxymethylphenyl)-1-ethanol, also known as salbutamol. The structure and synthetic plan of salbutamol are represented in Fig. 3.8.

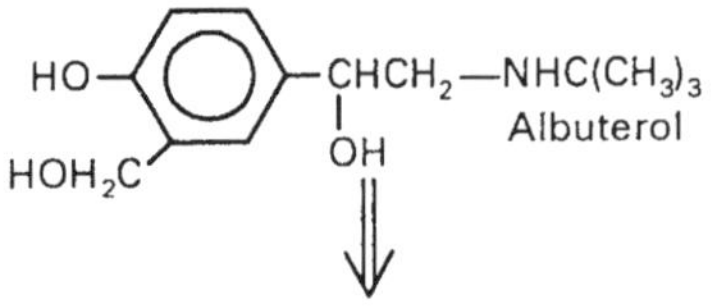

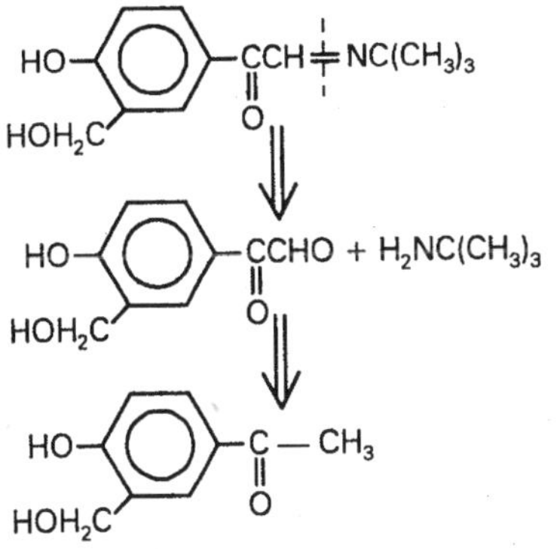

Fig. 3.8 *Structure and synthetic plan of salbutamol.*

Synthesis Salbutamol is synthesized from 4-hydroxy-3(hydroxymethyl) acetophenone. The synthesis sequentially involves: (i) bromination,

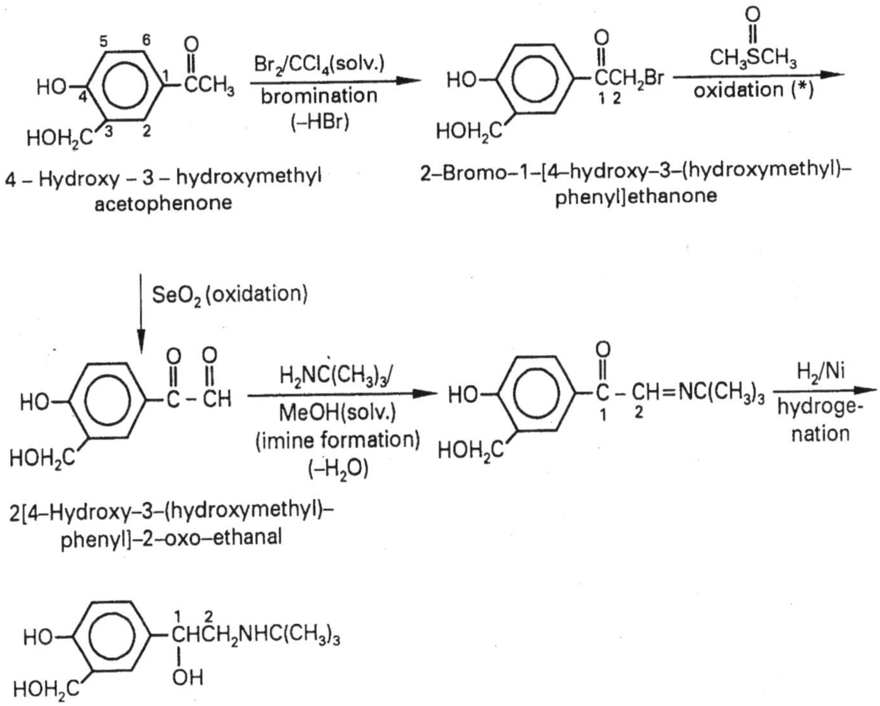

Scheme 3.8 Synthesis of salbutamol.

(ii) oxidation, (iii) the formation of an imine, and (iv) hydrogenation (Scheme 3.8).

Oxidation mechanism of 2-bromo-1-[4-hydroxy-3-(hydroxymethyl)-phenyl] ethanone with dimethylsulphoxide (DMSO).

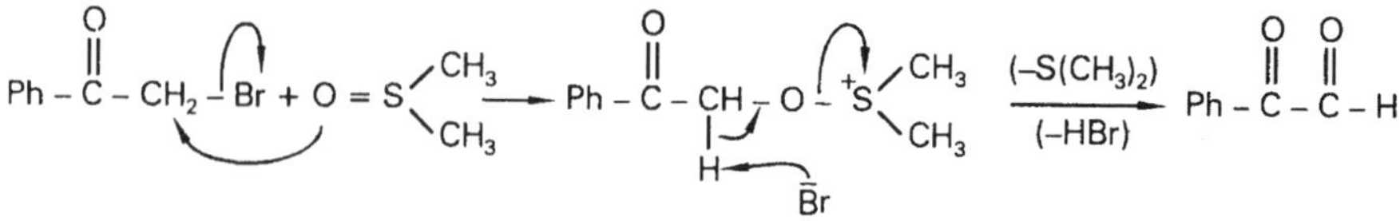

Therapeutic activity Salbutamol is a sympathomimetic (adrenergic) agent. It acts as a β-2 adrenergic receptor agonist situated in the bronchi. It inhibits bronchial spasms and is very effective in the treatment of bronchial asthma; it is a bronchodilator.

3.5.9 Analgin: a pentasubstituted five-membered heterocyclic compound

Analgin (novalgin) is sodium 1,5-dimethyl-(3-oxo-2-phenyl-2,3-dihydro-1H-4-pyrazo- loyl-(methyl)-aminomethane sulphonate. It is a derivative of pyrazole. Figure 3.9 depicts the structure and the synthetic plan of analgin.

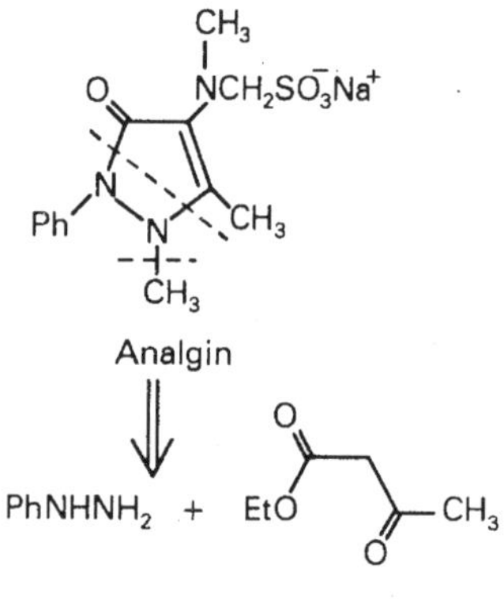

Fig. 3.9 *The structure and synthetic plan of analgin.*

Synthesis Analgin is synthesized from ethylacetoacetate (EAA) and involves a multi-step conversion. In the first step, a pyrazolone ring is constructed using EAA and phenylhydrazine. The reaction involves condensation, followed by cyclization. The resulting compound is reacted with CH_3I to carry out N-methylation and then it is nitrosated. The nitrous group is reduced to an amino group using zinc, in the presence of acetic

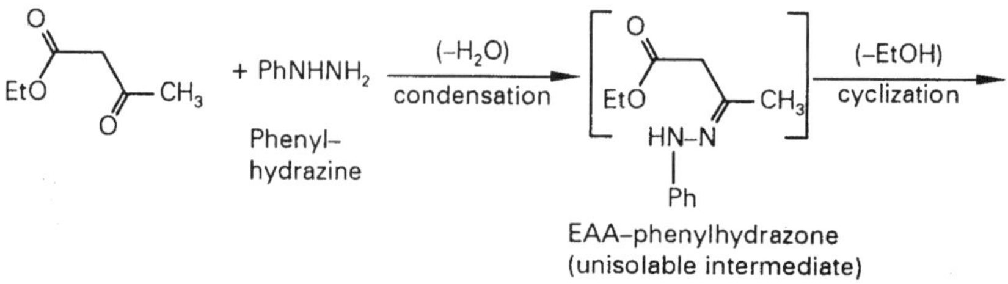

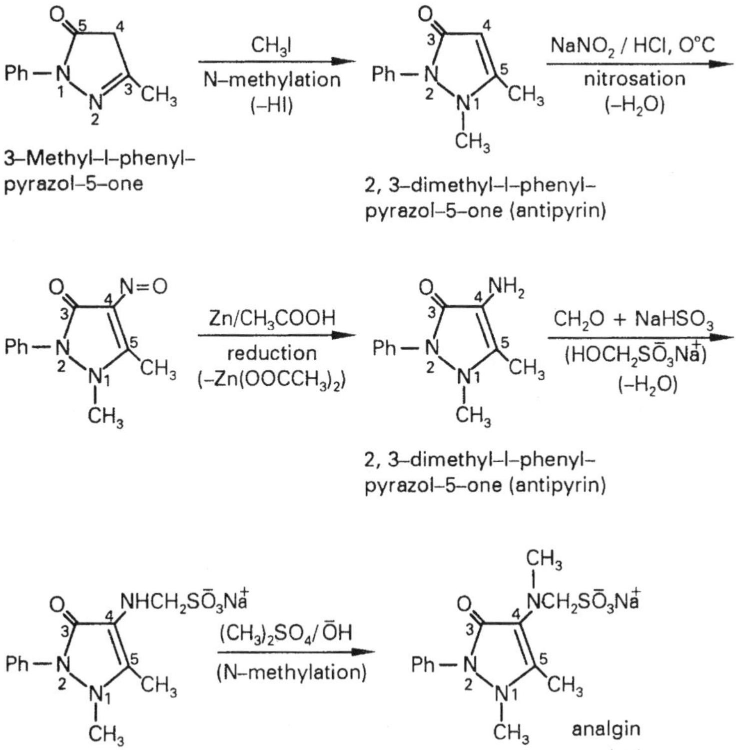

Scheme 3.9 Synthesis of analgin.

acid. The condensation of the amino group with formaldehyde in the presence of sodium bisulphite gives malubrin which, on N-methylation with dimethyl sulphate in a basic medium, gives analgin (Scheme 3.9).

Therapeutic activity Analgin is used as an antipyretic and an analgesic.

3.5.10 Metoclopramide: an anti-emetic drug

Metoclopramide is a tetrasubstituted benzene. The structure and guidelines for its synthesis are provided in Fig. 3.10.

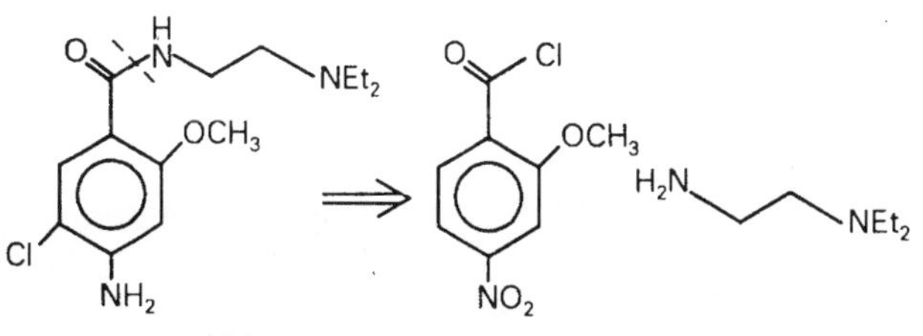

Fig. 3.10 *The structure and synthetic plan of metoclopramide.*

Synthesis It is synthesized from o-toludine and involves a multi-step conversion (Scheme 3.10).

Step 1 : The nitration of o-toluidine with nitric acid gives 2-methyl-5-nitroaniline. In this reaction, the methyl group acts as a p-directing group and the amino group acts as an m-directing group, due to protonation in the acid medium.

Step 2 : The amino group on diazotization, followed by acid hydrolysis, is converted into a hydroxyl group. The product is 2-methyl-5-nitrophenol.

Step 3 : The methylation of the phenolic compound with dimethyl sulphate in a basic medium gives the corresponding ether.

Step 4 : The oxidation of the product of Step 3 with potasium permanganate, followed by acidification, gives a benzoic acid derivative.

Step 5 : The carboxylic acid on treatment with thionyl chloride gives the corresponding acid chloride.

Step 6 : The acid chloride undergoes condensation with the 1° amino group of the diamine to yield the corresponding amide.

Step 7 : In this step, the nitro group is reduced to an amino group with hydrogen, in the presence of Ni as a catalyst.

Step 8 : It involves the acetylation of the amino group using acetic anhydride

Step 9 : The chlorination of the product in Step 8 preferentially enters into para to the methoxy group.

Step 10 : This final step involves the deacetylation of the acetamido group, which takes place on heating with diluted mineral acid, and results in the formation of metoclopramide (Scheme 3.10).

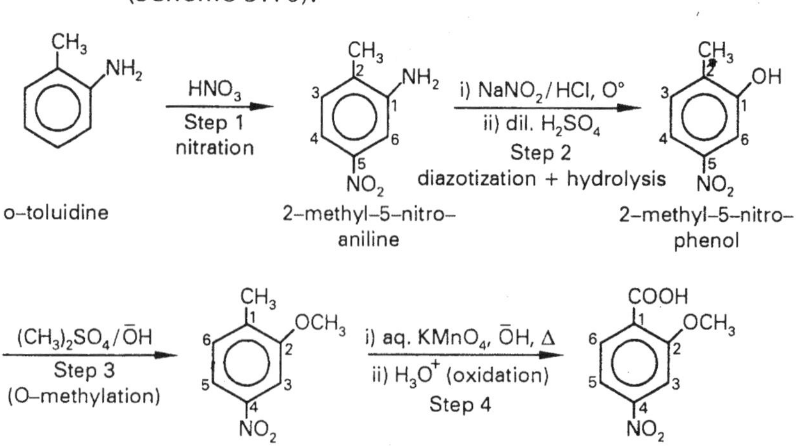

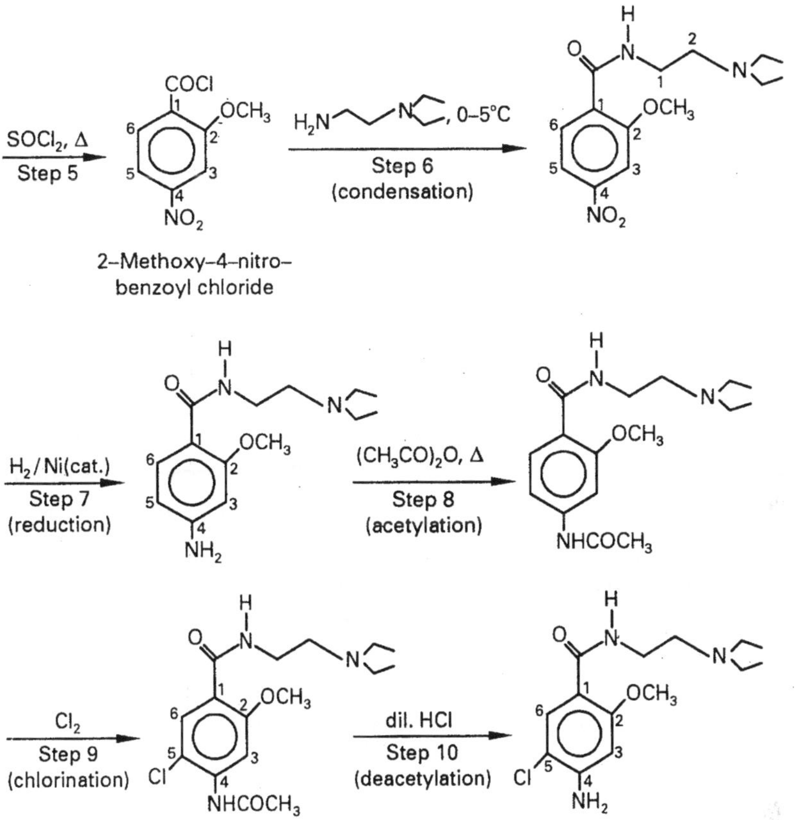

Scheme 3.10 Synthesis of metoclopramide.

Therapeutic activity It is used as an anti-emetic drug.

3.5.11 Chloroquine: an antimalarial drug

Chloroquine is a quinoline derivative. The structure and synthetic plan of the drug are presented in Fig. 3.11.

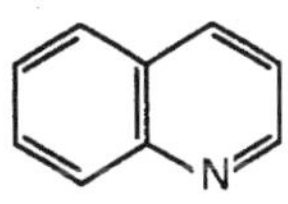

Quinoline

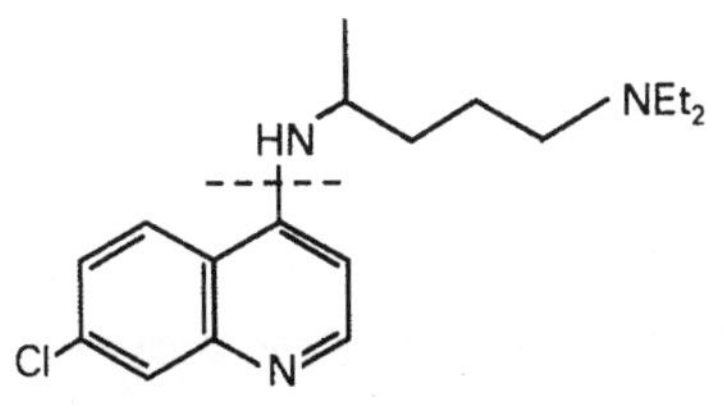

Chloroquine

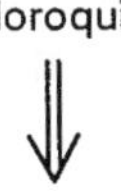

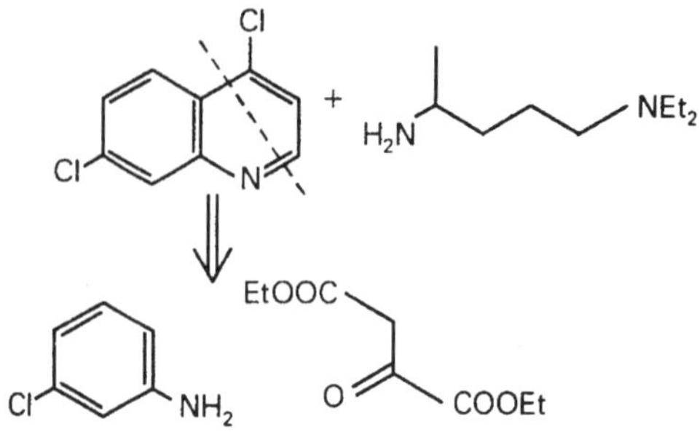

Fig. 3.11 *The structure and synthetic plan of chloroquine.*

Synthesis (Scheme 3.11) From the analyses of the structure of chloroquine, from the synthetic point of view, the essential reactants are 3-chloroaniline, diethyl 2-oxosuccinate and 2-amino-5-(diethylamino) pentane, respectively. 3-Chloroaniline undergoes condensation with diethyl 2-oxosuccinate to give an imine. The imine on heating in high boiling solvents loses a molecule of EtOH, leading to cyclization. In the subsequent step, saponification yields the corresponding carboxylic acid on treatment with dil. HCl. Heating the carboxylic acid at higher temperatures leads to decarboxylation, and subsequent treatment with phosphorous oxychloride results in the formation of a dichloroquinoline. The 'Cl' group present in the pyridine ring of quinoline undergoes nucleophilic substitution(S_NAr) with the diamine to produce chloroquine.

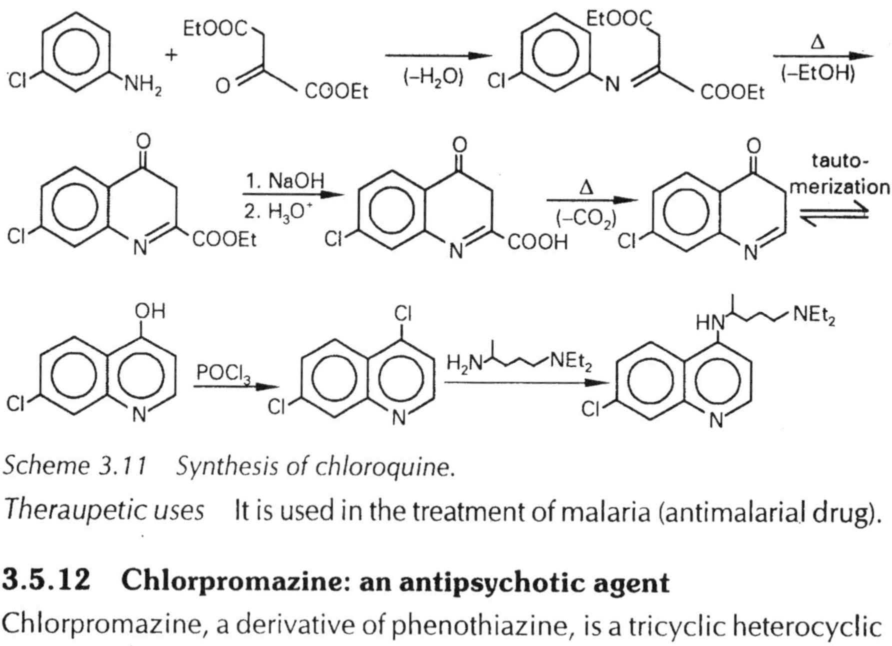

Scheme 3.11 Synthesis of chloroquine.

Theraupetic uses It is used in the treatment of malaria (antimalarial drug).

3.5.12 Chlorpromazine: an antipsychotic agent

Chlorpromazine, a derivative of phenothiazine, is a tricyclic heterocyclic compound. Its structure and synthetic plan are presented in Fig. 3.12.

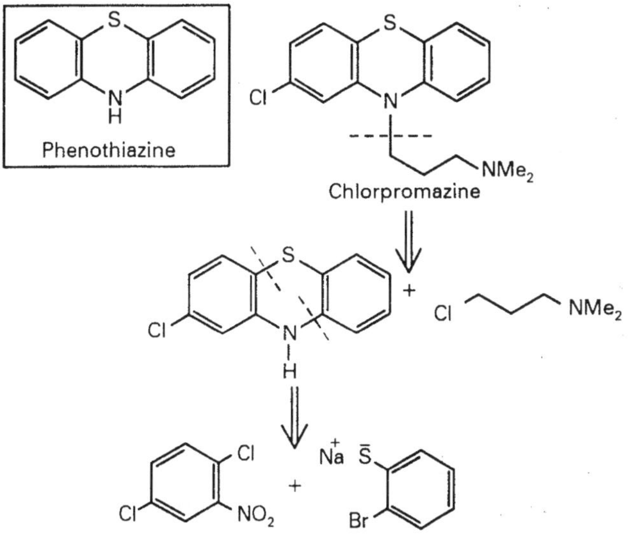

Fig. 3.12 *The structure and synthetic plan of chlorpromazine.*

Synthesis (Scheme 3.12) The required reactants are 2, 5-dichloronitrobenzene, sodium 2-bromo- thiophenoxide, and 3-chloro-N, N-dimethyl-1-propanamine. The chlorine at the 2 position of 1, 4-dichloro-2-nitrobenzene, is an activated group towards nucleophilic substitution. When it reacts with sodium 2-bromo thiophenoxide, the corresponding thioether is formed. The reduction of the nitro group yields an amino group. Ring closure (cyclization) of the amino compound to chloro-

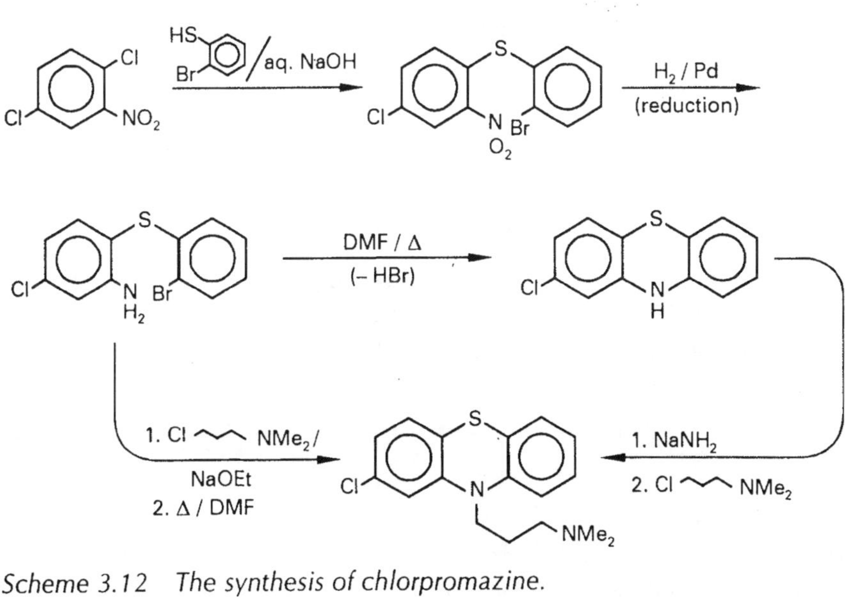

Scheme 3.12 *The synthesis of chlorpromazine.*

thiophenazine is achieved by heating it in the presence of dimethyl formamide (DMF) as a solvent. This step involves the removal of HBr. The side-chain attachment involves the alkylation of 'N' with 3-chloro-N, N-dimethyl-1-propanamine in a basic medium. Alternatively, the amino compound is alkylated first, followed by cyclization.

Therapeutic uses The efficacy of chlorpromazine and its many analogues led to a revolution in the management of mental disorders such as schizophrenia, psychotic depression and mania. It is now recognized that this class of drugs act as a dopamine antagonist by binding to the receptors for this neurotransmitter. It is also used for the prevention and treatment of nausea and vomiting.

3.5.13 Phenobarbital: a barbiturate

Barbituric acid is systematically known as hexahydro-2, 4, 6-pyrimidinetriones. Barbutirates are derivatives of barbituric acid. Phenobarbital is 5-ethyl-5-phenylhexahydro-2, 4, 6-pyrimidinetrione (5-ethyl-5-phenylbarbituric acid). The general structure and synthetic plan of barbiturates is shown in Fig. 3.13.

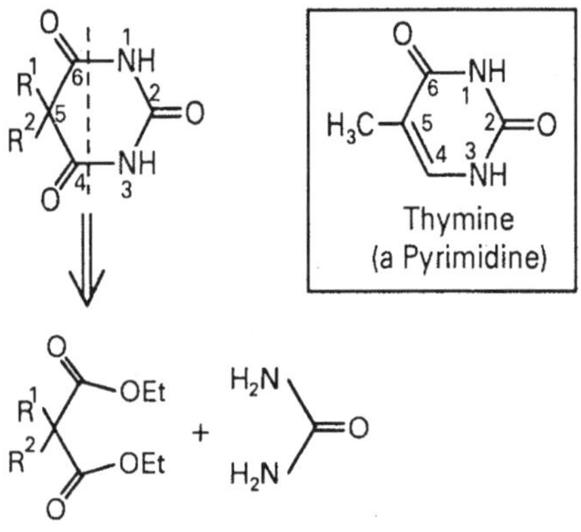

Fig. 3.13 *The structure and synthetic plan of barbiturates.*

An analysis of the structure of barbiturates, from the synthetic point of view, indicates that malonic ester or substituted malonic esters and urea are the starting materials. The condensation of these reactants is a base catalyzed reaction (Scheme 3.13).

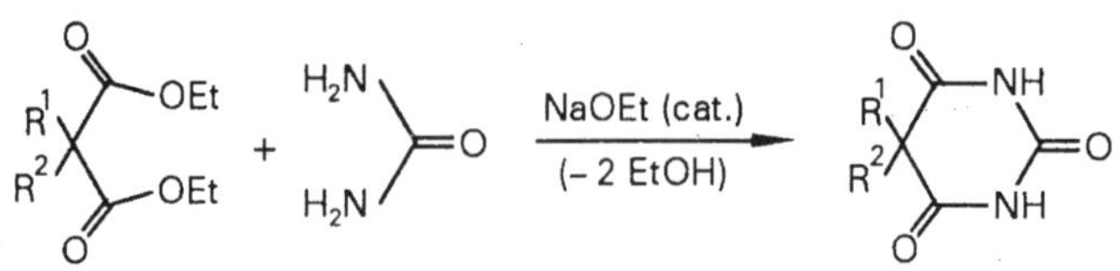

Scheme 3.13 Synthesis of barbiturates.

Some barbiturates are listed in Table 3.3.

Table 3.3 *Some Barbiturates*

R^1	R^2	**Barbituric acid Barbiturate**
H	H	Barbituric acid
Et	H	Barbital
Et	Et	Veronal
Et	Ph	Phenobarbital

Synthesis of phenobarbital (from phenyl acetic acid; Scheme 3.14) Ethyl phenyl malonic ester is difficult to prepare from malonic ester. For this reason, the malonic ester required for the synthesis of phenobarbital is made from phenyl acetic acid. When phenyl acetic acid is subjected to a reaction with $SOCl_2$, it is converted into the acid chloride which, on treatment with ethanol, gives the corresponding ester. One of the hydrogens of the methylene group of the ester is deprotonated using potassium t-butoxide as a base and then condensed with diethyl carbonate to give phenyl malonic ester. This intermediate is treated with sodium ethoxide to generate carbanion which is ethylated using ethyl chloride to produce ethyl phenyl malonic ester. This ester is condensed with urea in the presence of sodium ethoxide, as a catalyst, to yield phenobarbital.

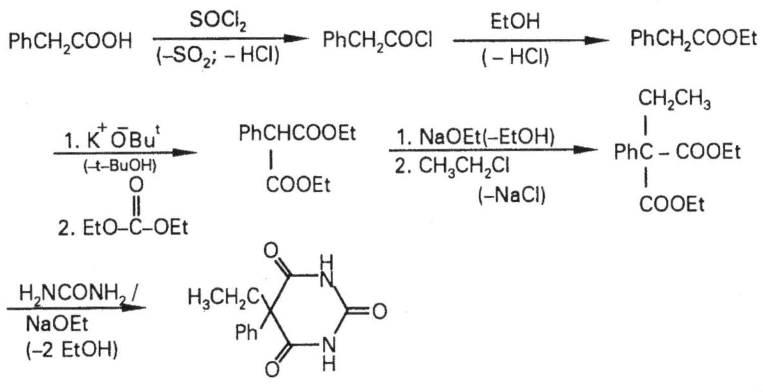

Scheme 3.14 The synthesis of phenobarbital starting from phenylacetic acid.

Therapeutic uses Barbiturates act on the Central Nervous System and are used as sedatives/hypnotics. Phenobarbital is an anticonvulsant and is effective in the management of epilepsy, in subhypnotic doses.

3.5.14 Omeprazole: an anti-ulcer drug

Omeprazole contains two heterocyclic moieties—benzimidazole and pyridine. The structure and synthetic plan of the drug are presented in Fig. 3.14.

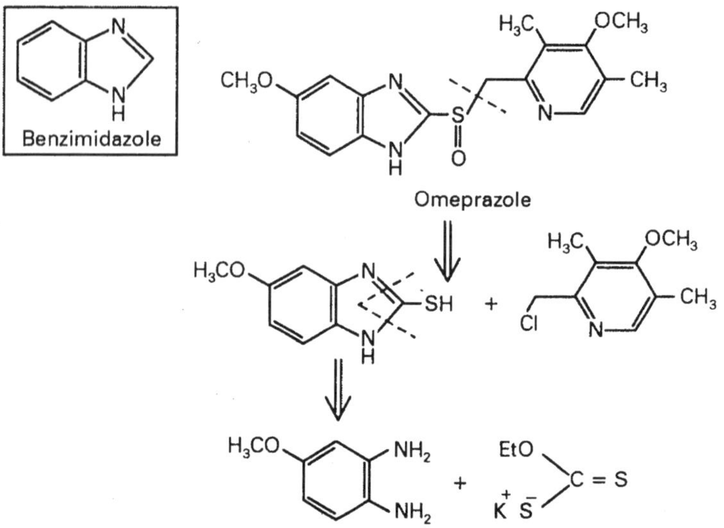

Fig. 3.14 *The structure and synthetic plan of omeprazole.*

Synthesis (Scheme 3.15) From the synthetic plan of omeprazole, three reactants are identified: i) 4-methoxybenzene-1,2-diamine known as 4-methoxy-o-phenylene diamine, ii) potassium ethylxanthate, and iii) a substituted pyridine. The synthesis of omeprazole involves the constructuction of an imidazole ring of benzimidazole, followed by a reaction with substituted chloromethyl pyridine. Methoxy o-phenylene diamine undergoes

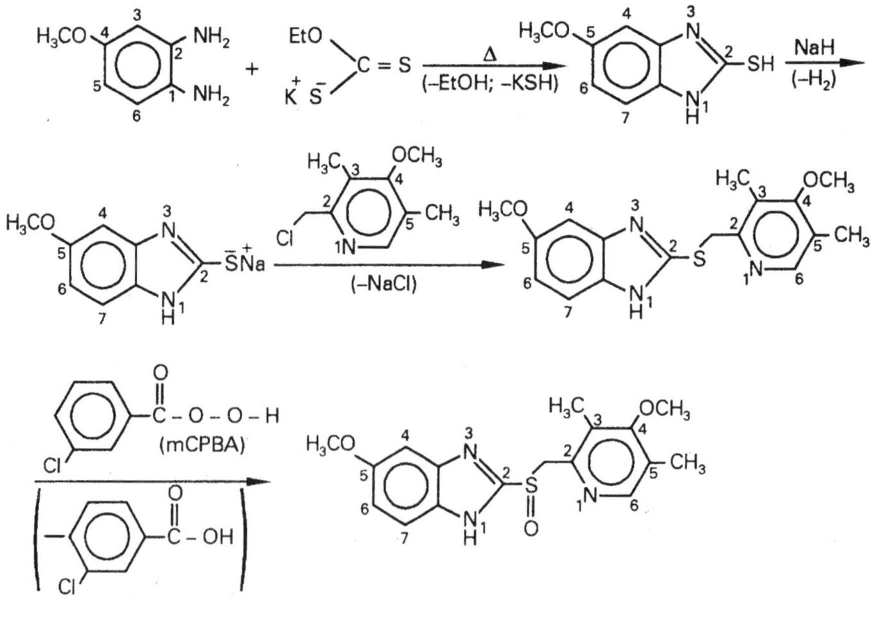

Scheme 3.15 The synthesis of omeprazole.

cyclization with potassium ethylxanthate to yield 5- methoxybenzimadazol-2-thiol. (Potassium ethylxanthate is prepared by the action of sodium ethoxide with carbon disulphide). The thiol group of this intermediate is converted into sodium salt, on treatment with NaH, which undergoes S_N2 reaction with a pyridine derivative to yield a thioether. The partial oxidation of sulphur with m-chloroperoxybenzoic acid (mCPBA) gives a sulphoxide, i.e., omeprazole.

Therapeutic uses The drug is useful for the treatment of ulcers (*anti-ulcer drug*). It acts directly on the stomach by inhibiting H^+, K^+ ATPase, which is responsible for acid secretion. It is an antisecretory agent.

3.5.15 Nifedipine: a drug for the treatment of angina and hypertension

Nifedipine is a 1, 4-dihydropyridine derivative. Its structure and synthetic plan are presented in Fig. 3.15.

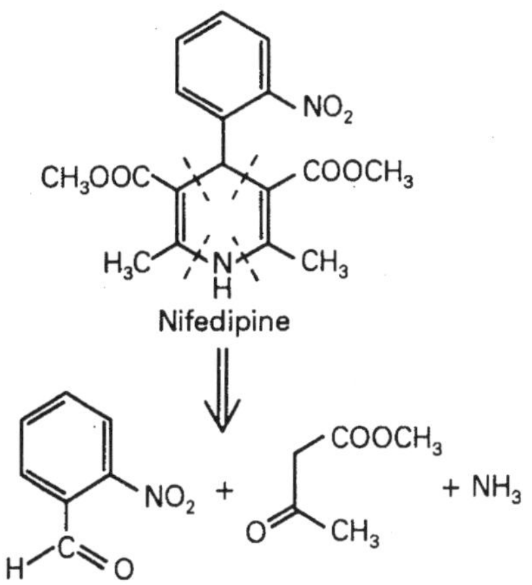

Fig. 3.15 *The structure and synthetic plan of nifedipine.*

Synthesis (Scheme 3.16) The synthesis of nifedipine is based on the classical Hantz pyridine synthesis. The net reaction for the synthesis of nifedipine involves one mole of o-nitrobenzaldehyde, two moles of methyl acetoacetate and one mole of NH_3 (Scheme 3.16). The mechanism of the formation of nifedipine is shown in Scheme 3.17.

Heating o-nitrobenzaldehyde with methyl acetoacetate in the presence of ammonia gives an unisolable intermediate, a benzylidine derivative. The reaction involves crossed aldol condensation. The intermediate, in turn, reacts with the second mole of methyl acetoacetate to give another unisolable intermediate, a 1, 5-diketone. The reaction of the dione with NH_3 involves cyclization, leading to the formation of nifedipine (Scheme 3.17).

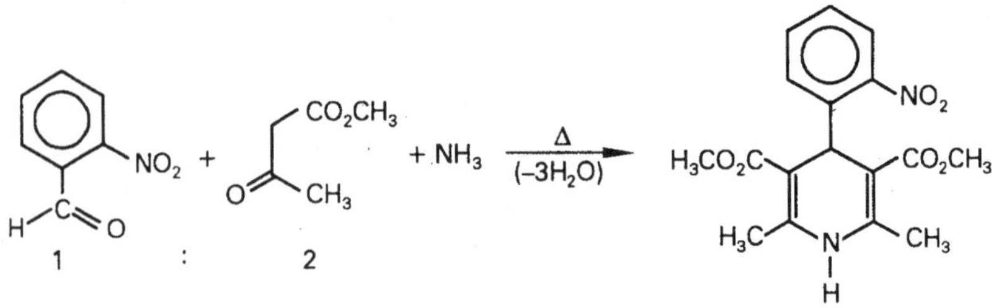

Scheme 3.16 The synthesis of nifedipine

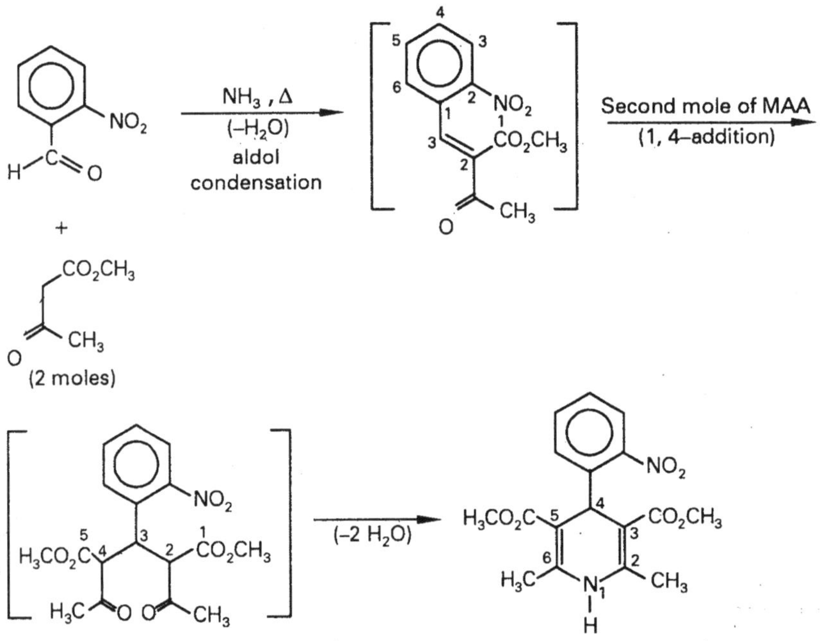

Scheme 3.17 Mechanism of the formation of nifedipine.

Therapeutic uses It is used in the treatment of angina and hypertension.

3.5.16 Ciprofloxacin: an antibacterial drug

The structure of ciprofloxacin contains a quinoline ring. Its structure and synthetic plan are shown in Fig. 3.16.

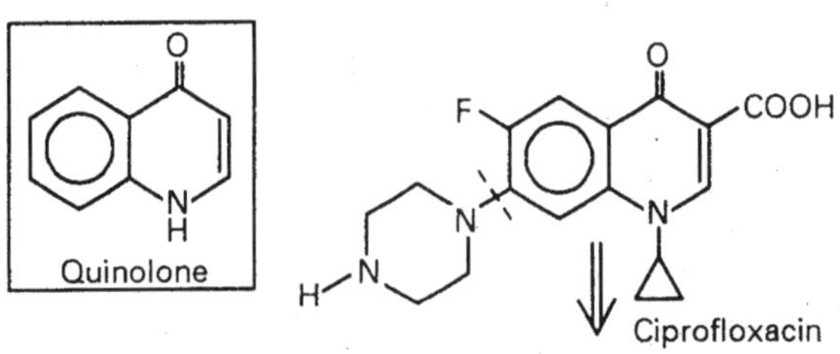

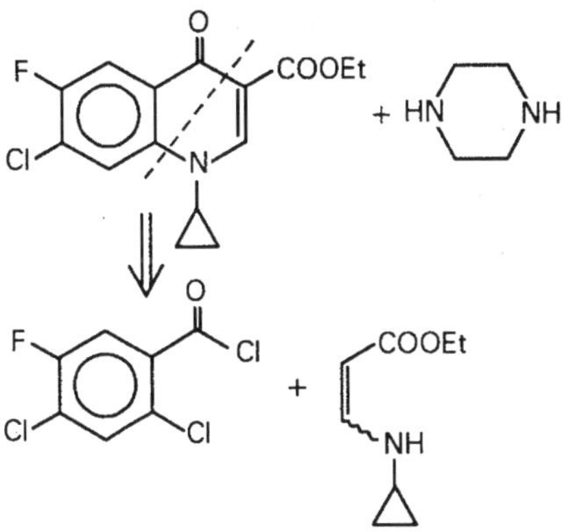

Fig. 3.16 *The structure and synthetic plan of ciprofloxacin.*

Synthesis (Scheme 3.18) From the synthetic plan, it is evident that the starting compounds for the synthesis of ciprofloxacin are a benzoyl chloride and an enamine. The enamine is condensed with the benzoyl derivative to yield a product, which is subsequently cyclized, using sodium hydride for the construction of a pyridine ring. The cyclized product is heated with pyrazine so that the chlorine group of the benzene is substituted (S_NAr). In the final step, the ester group is hydrolyzed to give ciprofloxacin (Scheme 3.18).

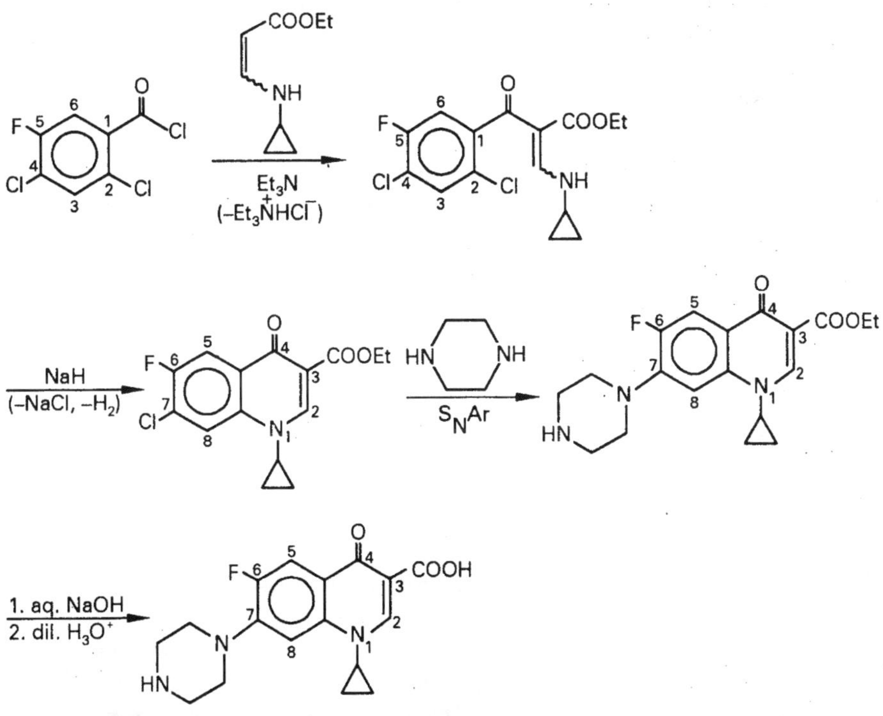

Scheme 3.18 The synthesis of ciprofloxacin.

Therapeutic use Ciprofloxacin is used as an antibacterial drug.

3.6 Natural drugs

3.6.1 Penicillin: a group of antibiotics

Discovery One of the most important discoveries in the 20th century was the discovery of penicillin—a group of antibiotics. An antibiotic is a substance produced by microorganisms (mould or bacterium) that resists the growth of, and even destroys, other microorganisms. Penicillin was discovered in 1928 by Alexander Flemming, an English bacteriologist. The discovery of penicillin was accidental and is an example of serendipity in science. Flemming was working on bacteria known to be pathogenic (disease causing), such as *Staphylococus aureus.* This germ causes boils and other types of infections. Before he went on vacation for a week, he left the culture in a petri dish at room temperature, instead of keeping it in the incubator. When he returned, he found that the mould, *Penicillium notatum,* had grown in the petri dish and he also found that the bacteria had been killed. Flemming was able to collect crude extracts of the active ingredient responsible for antibacterial action and named it penicillin (it branches out in the shape of a pencil, hence the name penicillin). The extracts were further purified and improved by Howard Florey and Ernst Boris Chain. These three scientists shared the Nobel Prize in 1945 for their great contribution to physiology and medicine.

Structures The term 'penicillins' does not represent a single compound, but a group of compounds with closely related structures. Structurally, penicillin consists of a β-lactam ring fused onto a thiazolidine ring. The general structure of penicillin, along with specific examples, is given in Fig. 3.17.

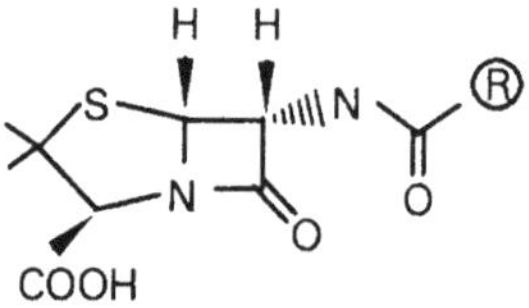

General Structure of Penicillins

Ⓡ = — CH_2Ph (Penicillin G)
Ⓡ = — OCH_2Ph (Penicillin V)
Ⓡ = — $CH_2-S-CH_2CH=CH_2$; (Penicillin O)

Fig. 3.17 *The structures of some penicillin drugs.*

Penicillin's mechanism of action is now well known. Penicillin prevents the synthesis of cell-walls by certain bacteria and causes their death. *All penicillins are bactericidal.* The cell-walls of bacteria are made up of mucoproteins (polymers of amino sugars and proteins). At the molecular level, penicillin inhibits an active enzyme of bacteria, *peptidoglycan transpeptidase*, which is responsible for the construction of the cell wall, in which the amino group of the enzyme opens up the β-lactam ring of penicillin making the enzyme inactive. Penicillin does not harm human cells. However, penicillin G and V have possible allergic reactions and other side effects in some people.

Before penicillin was discovered, many people died of blood poisoning, pneumonia, and other infectious diseases. Such deaths are now rare with the usage of penicillin, but some bacteria have developed resistance in the course of time. Now, penicillin is partially replaced by structurally related compounds known as *cephalosporins* (e.g., Cephalexin).

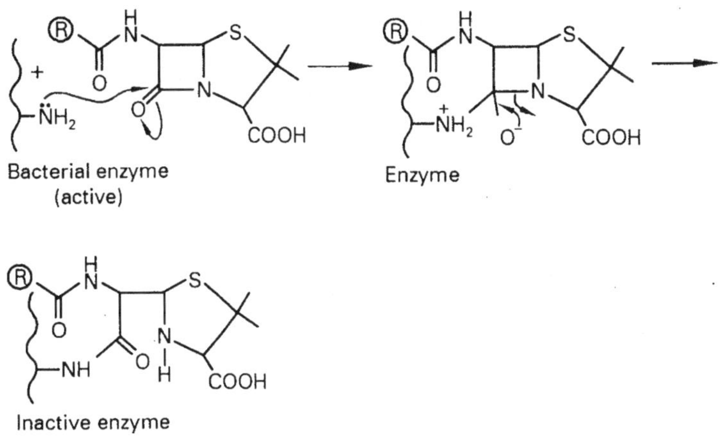

Fig. 3.18 *Mechanism of inactivation of enzyme of bacteria by penicillin.*

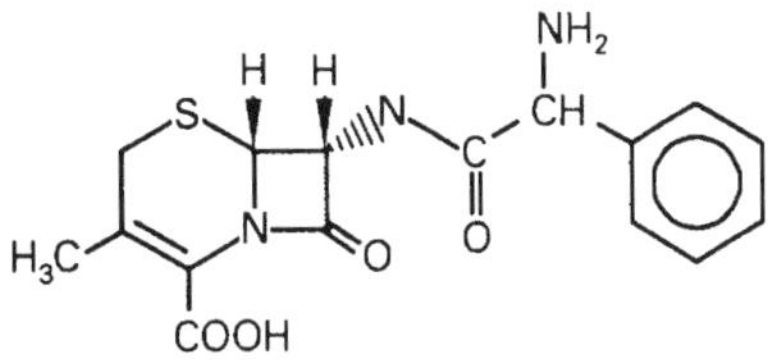

Cephalexin

In recent times, several semi-synthetic penicillins are being used as antibacterials. The fermentation of *Penicillinium chrysogenum* produces

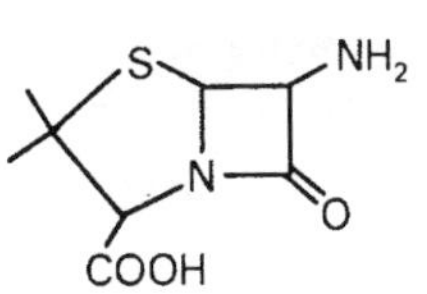

Penicillamine

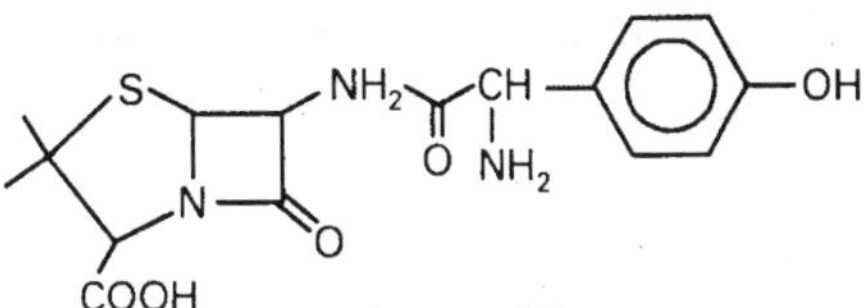

Amoxycillin

penicillamine. The chemical reaction of penicillamine with D-phenylglycine and p-hydroxy-D-phenylglycine, produces ampicillin and amoxycillin, respectively. Amoxycillin is the world's highest-selling antibiotic drug.

3.6.2 Production and isolation of penicillin

Penicillin is manufactured by aerobic fermentation. The source organism for this process was, initially *Penicillium notatum*. But now *Penicillium chrysogenum* is used because it produces higher yield of penicillin. Corn steep liquor is used as a fermentation medium and it consists of various ingredients as shown in Table 3.4.

Table 3.4 *Ingredients for Penicillin Synthesis by Fermentation*

Type of Ingredients	Specific Ingredients (%)
Main carbohydrate	Lactose, 3.0–4.0
Other carbohydrates	Glucose, 0–0.5 and Polysaccharides
Organic acids	Acetic, ~ 0.05, Lactic, ~ 0.5
Special precursors	Phenylethylamine
Main N source	Amines, amino acids, peptides
Other N source	Ammonia

Production and isolation of penicillin G: Step-by-step description of various stages

1. Spores of *Penicillium chrysogenum* are used to inoculate the medium in a flask.
2. **Shaker flask** The flask is incubated for 4-days on a shaker at 25°C.
3. **Transfer vessel** The contents of the flask is transferred into a medium and incubated at 25°C.
4. **Seed tank** (reactor) The contents of the transfer vessel are passed into a stainless steel tank and incubated for 3 days.
5. **Fermentation tank** The contents of the reactor is transformed into a medium in a fermentor and incubated for 5–6 days to produce penicillin.
6. **Rotary filter** The contents of the fermentation vessel is filtered.
7. **Extractors** The filtrate is passed into a series of extractors, wherein penicillin is extracted into amyl alcohol.
8. **Vacuum still** The crystallization of penicillin takes place here.
9. Penicillin is extracted into aq.phosphate buffer from amyl acetate and filtered and crystallized (from butanol-water mixture and converted into potassium salt or procaine salt).
10. **Vacuum drier** Penicillin G is freed from solvent impurities.

Table 3.5 *Names of Synthetic Drugs, Starting Compound for Synthesis and their Therapeutic Uses*

Name of the drug	Starting Compound	Therapeutic uses
1. Sulphanilamide[1]	Aniline/chlorobenzene	Bacteriostatic drug
2. Paracetamol[2]	Phenol/ p-nitrochlorobenzene	Antipyretic/Analgesic
3. Aspirin[2]	Salicyclic acid	Antipyretic/Analgesic
4. Oil of wintergreen	Salicylic acid	Treatment of lumbago, and sciatica
5. Mephensin[2]	o-Cresol	Potent muscle relaxant
6. Ibuprofen[2]	Isobutyl benzene	Anti-inflammatory agent
7. L-Dopa[2]	3,4-dihydroxybenzaldehyde and N-acetylglycine	Antiparkinsonian drug
8. Albuterol[2] (salbutamol)	4-hydroxy-3-hydroxymethyl-acetophenone	Bronchodilating agent (treatment of bronchial asthma)
9. Analgin[2]	Ethyl acetoacetate and phenylhydrazine	Antipyretic/Analgesic
10. Metoclopramide[2]	o-toludine	Anti-emetic drug
11. Chloroquine[1]	3-Chloroaniline and diethyl oxoglutarate	Antimalarial
12. Chlorpromazine[2]	2,4-dichloronitrobenzene and o-bromobenzenethiol	Treatment of mental disorders such as schizophrenia, psychotic depression, mania
13. Phenobarbital[2]	Phenyl acetic acid	Sedative/hypnotic
14. Omeprazole[2]	4-methoxybenzene-1, 2-diamine	Anti-ulcer drug
15. Nifedipine[2]	o-nitrobenzaldehyde and methylacetoacetate	Angina and hypertension
16. Ciprofloxacin[1]	2,4-dichloro-5-fluoro-benzoyl chloride	Antibacterial agent

[1]Chemotherapeutic agent [2]Pharmocodynamic agent

QUESTIONS

1. What are vitamins? How are they classified? Mention two examples of each type. Draw the structures of any two vitamins.
2. Mention the names of any three vitamins and, their major physiological functions, the diseases caused due to deficiency, and their natural sources.

3. What are hormones? Give the names of two hormones, draw the structure of one of the hormones you have mentioned and indicate its physiological effects.
4. How are the following drugs synthesized in the laboratory? (Write the chemical equations.)
   i) Sulphanilamide (from aniline)
   ii) Aspirin (from phenol)
   iii) Paracetamol (from p-nitrochlorobenzene)
5. How is metoclopramide synthesized from o-toludine? (Write the chemical equations involved.)
6. How would you accomplish the synthesis of the following drugs in the laboratory? (Write the chemical equations.)
   i) Mephensin (from o-cresol)
   ii) Salbutamol (from 4-hydroxy-(3-hydroxymethyl)-acetophenone)
7. How would you accomplish the synthesis of analgin from ethylacetoacetate ? (Write the chemical equations involved).
8. Mention the names of two drugs you have studied, that consists of one chiral carbon in their structure, and draw their stereochemical formulae. Write the chemical equation for synthesis of one of such drugs from suitable starting materials.
9. Draw the stereochemical formulae for: (i) L-Dopa (Fisher projection), (ii) therapeutically active form of Ibuprofen (wedge-dash wedge-line formula). Formulate the synthesis of Ibuprofen (racemic mixture) from 4-isobutylacetophenone (write the chemical equation involved).
10. What are antibiotics? Write a note on the discovery of penicillin. Draw the structures of penicillin G and V. Give an example of an antibiotic which is structurally related to the penicillin group of antibiotics which are the most widely used drugs.
11. Draw the structures of penicillin G and V and write a note on the isolation of penicillin.
12. Formulate the synthesis of a) Chloroquine (from 3-chloroaniline) b) Chloropromazine (from 1,4-dichloro-2-nitrobenzene)
13. What are barbiturates? Write the general structure of barbiturates. How would you synthesize phenobarbital from phenylacetic acid? (write the chemical equations.)
14. Provide the synthetic plan for nifedipine and ciprofloxacin and recognize the suitable starting materials.
15. Mention the therapeutic properties of: i) Chloroquine ii) Chloropromazine iii) Phenobarbital iv) Omeprazole v) Nifedipine vi) Ciprofloxacin.

Provide the synthetic plan for any one of them to recognize the suitable starting materials.

16. Distinguish between the following pairs of words and give an example for each one:
    i) antibacterial and antibiotic
    ii) analgesic and antipyretic
    iii) niacin and nausea
    iv) vitamins and hormones
    v) prodrug and drug
    vi) sulphanilamide and sulphonamide
17. Briefly explain the following and provide suitable reasons.
    i) Acetylsalicylic acid, in the intestine, hydrolyzes to salicylic acid—responsible for antipyretic and analgesic action. Why cannot salicylic acid be used as a drug directly?
    ii) L-dopa, used as a drug, is decarboxylated in the body to produce dopamine—responsible for curing Parkinson's disease. Why is it that dopamine not used as a drug directly?
    iii) Milk is supplemented with Vitamin D in most of the cold countries (where less sunlight is available).
    iv) Not all hormones are steroids.
    v) Vitamins A, D, E and K are fat-soluble, whereas vitamins of the B and C group are water-soluble.
    vi) Vitamin D_2 is often called the "sunshine vitamin".
    vii) Sulphanilamide is a bacteriostatic, but not a bactericidal, drug.
18. Compare and contrast the therapeutic properties of the following pairs of drugs:
    i) Aspirin and Paracetamol
    ii) Ibuprofen and Aspirin
    iii) Sulphanilamide and Penicillin
19. Explain the mechanism of action of the following drugs briefly in relation to their therapeutic properties mentioned against each one.
    i) Sulphanilamide - *antibacterial*
    ii) Aspirin - *analgesic activity*
    iii) Ibuprofen - *anti-inflammatory*
    iv) L-Dopa - *antiparkinsonian drug*
    v) Penicillin G - *antibiotic activity*
20. State whether the following statements are *True* or *False*.
    i) Carrots contain Vitamin A (retinol).

ii) Vitamins are produced in the human body, whereas hormones are not.

iii) Nicotinamide (niacin, vitamin B_3) is a part of coenzymes NAD (Nicotinamide Adenine Dinucleotide) and NADP (Nicotinamide Adenine Dinucleotide Phosphate).

iv) All vitamins contain an amino group.

v) Male sex hormones are called androgens and female sex hormones are called esterogens.

vi) Vitamins and hormones can be considered as drugs.

vii) D-Dopa can also be used as a drug.

viii) Sulpha drugs were extensively used during World War II to prevent infections in wounds.

ix) The term 'penicillin' represents a specific example of an antibiotic drug.

x) Aspirin, Paracetamol and Analgin are examples of antipyretic and analgesic drugs.

21. Fill in the following blanks with the suitable answers.

i) Anemia is caused due to a deficiency of ____________ (vitamin).

ii) Enols are generally less stable. They tautomerize to an aldehyde or a ketone. An example of a vitamin which possesses stable enolic structure is ________.

iii) Insulin, secreted by pancreas, is an example of a ________ ________ (vitamin/hormone).

iv) Pyridoxal, one of the constituents of vitamin B_6, has the following structure:

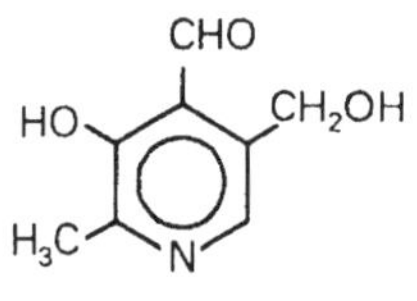

The structures of pyridoxol and pyridoxamine are ___________ and ________________, respectively.

v) Chlorosulphonation of chlorobenzene, followed by ammonolysis gives ______________ (MF = $C_6H_8N_2O_2S$).

vi) Acetylation of p-aminophenol with Ac_2O in AcOH gives ____________ (a drug).

vii) Methyl salicylate is commonly known as _______________.

viii) In terms of R/S configuration, L-Dopa corresponds to _____________.

ix) The other name for albuterol is ____________.

22. Match the vitamins in column I with the deficiency diseases (randomly placed) mentioned in column II.

	Column I			Column II
i)	Retinol	( )	a)	Rickets
ii)	Cobalamine	( )	b)	Scurvy
iii)	Ascorbic acid	( )	c)	Hemorrhage
iv)	Calciferol	( )	d)	Night blindness
v)	a-Tocopherol	( )	e)	Pernicious anemia
vi)	Phylloquinone	( )	f)	Sterility; muscular dystrophy

23. Match the drugs given in Column I and therapeutic uses in Column II.

	Column I			Column II
i)	Paracetamol	( )	a)	Anti-emetic
ii)	Mephensin	( )	b)	Antibiotic
iii)	Albuterol	( )	c)	Antipyretic and analgesic
iv)	Metoclopramide	( )	d)	Bronchial asthma
v)	Penicillin G	( )	e)	Muscle relaxant

Answers to selected questions

17. i) Salicylic acid is sour and causes irritation when taken orally, whereas aspirin does not cause such side effects. For this reason, salicylic acid is not used directly as a drug.

ii) Dopamine itself cannot be used as a drug directly because it cannot penetrate into the cerebral fluid (of the brain) from the bloodstream. L-Dopa (structurally related to L-tyrosine, an amino acid) can enter the cerebral fluid where it is converted into dopamine.

iii) In cold countries people may not be sufficiently exposed to sunlight, necessary for the conversion of ergosterol into calciferol (vitamin D_2) in the body. As a result, this vitamin may not be sufficiently synthesized. Therefore, milk is supplemented with the vitamin to overcome any deficiency.

iv) Some of the steroids function as hormones and are called steroidal hormones (e.g., testosterone). There are also some hormones which are structurally related to amino acids and, proteins (e.g., insulin). For this reason, all hormones are not steroids.

v) Structurally, vitamins A, D, E and K consist of more hydrocarbon and less polar groups. On the whole, these vitamins are less polar and soluble in less polar medium i.e., fats. The B group of vitamins and Vitamin C are more polar and hence soluble in a higher polar medium, i.e., water.

vi) Sulphanilamide is a drug which inhibits the growth of bacteria, but does not destroy them. Therefore, it is bacteriostatic but not bactericidal.

20. i) False ii) False iii) True iv) False
v) True vi) True vii) False viii) True
ix) False x) True

21. i) Folic acid
ii) Ascorbic acid
iii) Hormone

iv) 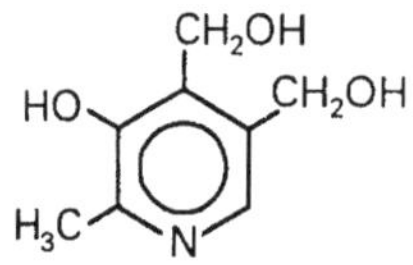

and 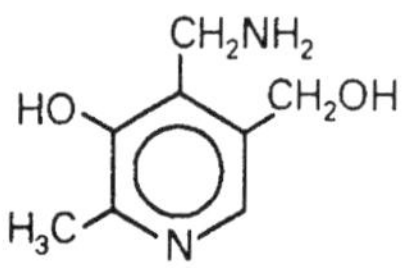

v) Sulphanilamide (4-aminobenzenesulphonamide)
vi) Paracetamol (acetaminophen)
vii) vii) Oil of wintergreen
viii) (S)-Dopa
ix) Salbutamol

22. i) (d)
ii) (e)
iii) (b)
iv) (a)
v) (f)
vi) (c)

23) i) (c)
ii) (e)
iii) (d)
iv) (a)
v) (b)

Appendix

Vitamin B_{12} (Cobalamin): The vitamin with the largest molecular structure and co-containing complex

Structural features The vitamin B_{12} has the largest molecular structure, and is the only vitamin which is a coordinate complex(octahedral) containing cobalt as a metal ion. The name, *cobalamin,* is derived from the inclusion of cobalt in its structure. This makes vitamin B_{12} unique among vitamins, in addition to other factors. It is the first natural product that was found to contain cobalt.

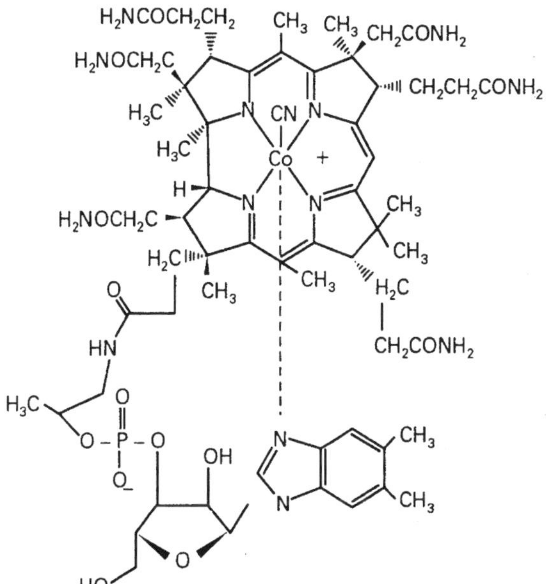

Vitamin B_{12}

The structure of vitamin B_{12} has been well established through physical (including spectroscopic) and chemical methods. The structure involves various parts: (a) benzimidazole moiety (b) benzimidazole-a-ribofuranoside (c) phosphate group (d) corrin moiety (B_{12} is a corrinoid) (e) Co as a central metal ion: **Cyanocobalamin** consists of CN group bonded to cobalt.

Biochemical functions Vitamin B_{12} is necessary for performing various important biochemical functions. It is a coenzyme in the reduction of ribonucleotide to deoxyribonuclotide. It catalyzes the synthesis of nucleic acids, RBC and WBC, and maintains the reproductive and nervous systems.

Deficiency effects and sources The deficiency of this vitamin causes poor cell-division and pernicious anemia (characterized by abnormally large RBC). The vitamin occurs only in animals and microorganisms. The major sources of the vitamin are liver, egg and fish and liver extract. The daily recommended intake in adults is 3–4 mg. People, who do not consume milk, eggs and other animal products may suffer from this deficiency. They are advised to supplement their diet with this vitamin, as it is not found in vegetables.

Vitamin B_{12} is commercially produced by the fermentation of *the streptomyces* species.

4 FORMULATION OF DRUGS

4.1 *Introduction*

The study of the conversion of drug into a **medicine** (the design of dosage forms or formulations) and its manufacture, stability and the effectiveness of the drug dosage form is termed as **pharmaceutics.**

There are three important stages in the use of a drug as a medicine, i.e., the conversion of a drug into a formulation: 1) the discovery of the drug, 2) the manufacture of the drug in bulk form (bulk drug manufacture), and 3) the formulation of a drug into different dosage forms like tablet, capsule, injection, syrup, cream, etc. The discoverer of the drug conducts extensive clinical trials of the new drug with respect to: 1) the physiochemical properties of the drug, like aqueous solubility, partition coefficient in biological membranes of proteins and lipids, dissolution rate, physical form and stability; 2) biopharmaceutical considerations, such as how the route of administration of a dosage form affects the rate and extent of drug absorption into the body; 3) therapeutic considerations of the disease state to be treated which, in turn, decides the most suitable type of dosage form, dose frequency, possible routes of administration, onset time, duration of action and intensity of action of the drug to be used.

4.2 *Need for the conversion of drugs into medicine (formulations)*

Drugs are rarely administered solely as pure chemical substances, but are always given in formulated preparations for the following reasons.

1. A single dose of many drugs is in the milligram range, from about 0.25 to 250 mg. It is very difficult to weigh and handle such a small quantity accurately and also it is very difficult to swallow such small amounts of the drug.
2. Many drugs have a bitter taste and this results in poor compliance, particularly in the case of pediatric patients.
3. Many drugs have an unpleasant odour, flavour and colour.

4. When the drug is taken directly, it is absorbed in a small area in the gastrointestinal tract (GIT), leading to gastric irritation.
5. Several drugs have poor bioavailability when taken in the pure form.
6. Some drugs are very unstable in the highly acidic environment of the stomach (hydrolysis or degradation in the stomach). Hence, the enteral (oral) route of administration is to be avoided.
7. In several cases, the drug action must take place quickly. So, the drug has to be administered parenterally (directly into the systemic circulation in the form of injection).
8. The drug substance has to be protected from atmospheric oxygen and humidity.
9. Some drugs have to act slowly and continuously for several hours or days (sustained release or controlled release).
10. Some drugs have to be specifically delivered directly to certain organs (e.g., the lungs, by inhalation of the drug, i.e., as an aerosol spray).
11. Several patients (particularly the elderly) use many drugs simultaneously. These drugs should be in a readily identifiable form to avoid any confusion or misuse.

Many of the common drugs are organic compounds with poor solubility in water. For a drug to act, it should be sufficiently soluble in the intracellular and extracellular fluids of the body. Drugs that are basic in nature are converted into salts, such as hydrochloride or sulfate or maleate.

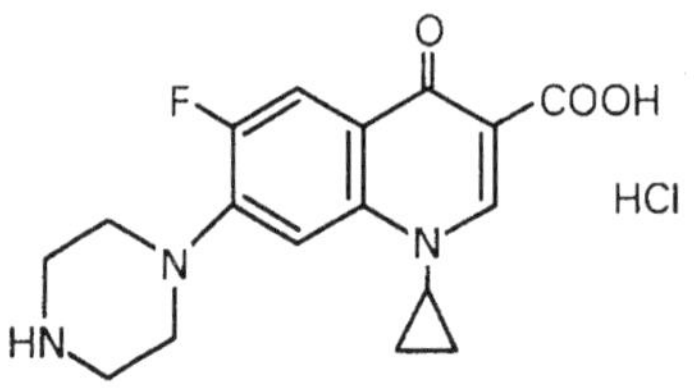

E.g. 1 Ciprofloxacin hydrochloride.

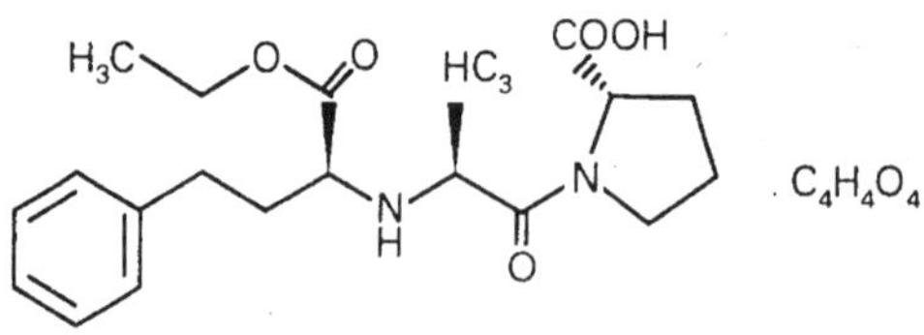

E.g. 2 Enalapril maleate

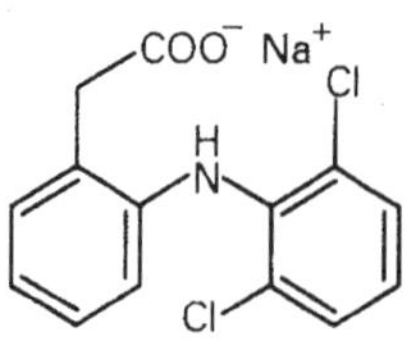

E.g. 3 Dichlofenac sodium

Drugs that are acidic in nature are converted into their sodium or potassium salts. The conversion of a drug into its salt greatly increases its solubility in water. Further, the salts have higher chemical stability. Drugs such as aspirin and paracetamol are highly water- soluble and hence need not be made into salts.

There are several conveniences when the pure drug is converted into a formulation, i.e., tablet, injection, syrup, etc.

1. There is a convenience in using the drug as its dosage form such as a tablet or capsule, to carry, to handle, to swallow; as a solution to be injected easily; and as a cream that can be readily applied to the skin.
2. Formulated drugs, like syrups, are readily administrable to pediatric patients.
3. The formulated drugs have an organoleptically amicable, i.e., aesthetic appearance, pleasant taste, good flavour, attractive and recognizable colour and shape.
4. Drug formulation has a better absorption in the gastrointestinal tract, greater bioavailability, and as the absorption of the drug takes place on a larger surface area, there is less gastric bleeding or irritation.
5. Drug delivery is faster when it is administered as an injection.
6. With the help of suitable additives and coatings, a drug can be delivered in a slow and controlled manner into the gastrointestinal tract.

Therefore, a drug has to be made into a suitable formulation, by using some solid or liquid non-therapeutic agents or additives. The additives used in drug formulations are known as pharmaceutical additives or adjuvants or excipients.

4.3 Additives and their role

In preparing different dosage forms (medicines) it is essential to add non-therapeutic agents called additives or excipients or adjuvants. Each of the additives has its specific role in the dosage form. All these additives are non-toxic and are known as permitted or official.

i. *Diluents* Diluents are usually finely-powdered, inert, solid substances that can be mixed with the medicaments (drugs) in order to bring up the weight of the dosage forms to the desired quantity. The diluents are used where the quantity of the medicament is small. The commonly used diluents are sugars: dextrose, lactose, sucrose, amylose, mannitol, sorbitol; polysaccharides: starches, microcrystalline cellulose, powdered cellulose; inorganic compounds: dibasic calcium phosphate, calcium lactate trihydrate, magnesium carbonate, etc.

ii. *Binders* Binding agents are used to impart cohesiveness to powdered particles and they give sufficient strength to the granules, so as to prevent them from crumbling. The properties of granules like uniformity of size, hardness, compressibility, etc., in turn, are intimately related to the nature and qualities of the binding agent used for the conversion of finely-powdered materials into granules. The commonly used binding agents are acacia, gum tragacanth, starch, gelatin, cellulose, sodium alginate, methylcellulose, ethylcellulose, etc.

iii. *Granulating agents* These agents are added to the therapeutic agent to convert finely-powdered particles into granules; e.g., water, alcohol, etc.

iv. *Disintegrants* Disintegrants are used in solid dosage forms. These substances are added to facilitate the disintegration of tablets in the gastrointestinal tract. Generally, three types of disintegrating agents are used in formulations. They are:

  a) Substances that swell on coming in contact with water; e.g., maize starch, potato starch, and methylcellulose.

  b) Substances that produce effervescence when they come in contact with water; e.g., citric acid, tartaric acid, and sodium carbonate.

  c) Substances that melt at body temperature; e.g., cocoa butter.

v. *Lubricants* Lubricants are added to reduce interparticular friction and to reduce the friction between the tablet and die wall—calcium stearate; magnesium stearate, talc etc.

vi. *Vehicle* A vehicle is a medium in which the ingredients of a formulation are dissolved, suspended or dispersed for their administration and rapid pharmaceutical action. They are used in formulating a variety of liquid dosage forms for oral and parenteral administration.

  Generally, oral liquids are aqueous preparations. Potential solutions for intravenous use are aqueous, whereas intramuscular injections may be aqueous or oleaginous. Aqueous vehicles are acacia syrup, aromatic syrup, cherry syrup, cocoa syrup, and orange syrup. Oleaginous vehicles are corn oil, mineral oil, peanut oil, sesame oil, etc. Sterile vehicles are bacterostatic sodium chloride injection, and bacterostatic water for injection.

vii. *Suspending agents* These are hydrophilic colloids that form colloidal dispersions with water and increase the viscosity of the continuous phase, so that the particle remains suspended throughout the vehicle in which they are not soluble. The resultant suspensions may be formulated for use orally, parenterally, opthalmically, topically, or by other routes. Some examples are gum acacia, tragacanth, starch, sodium alginate, cellulose derivatives, bentonite, and kaolin.

viii. *Stabilizing agents* The stability of a dosage form may refer to the stability of its chemical composition or immunity against microbial spoilage. These stability aspects can be overcome by adding additives like antioxidants, antimicrobial agents and antifungal agents.

   a) *Antioxidants* Antioxidants inhibit the oxidation of the dosage form and thus are used to prevent the deterioration of preparations by the oxidative process. For example, ascorbic acid, ascorbil palmitate, sodium ascorbate, sodium bisulphate, sodium metabisulphite, and butylated hydroxy anisole.

   b) *Antimicrobials* They are used in liquid and semi-solid preparations to prevent the growth of microorganisms; e.g., benzyl alcohol, phenol, phenyl ethyl alcohol, and chlorobutanol.

   c) *Antifungals* They are used in liquid and semi-solid preparations to prevent the growth of fungi; e.g., benzoic acid, butyl paraben, sodium benzoate, sodium propionate, and ethyl paraben.

ix. *Flavourants* Flavourants are used to impart a pleasant flavor and often odour to a pharmaceutical preparation. Generally, these substances are added to lozenges, effervescent tablets, chewable tablets, etc. Flavouring agents are generally volatile in nature; therefore, they must be sprayed over the granules before compression. For example, anise oil, lemon oil, cherry, menthol, orange oil, and peppermint are some of the commonly used flavouring agents.

x. *Sweeteners* These substances are added to formulations to impart a sweet taste to tablets; e.g., mannitol, dextrose, saccharin sodium, aspartame, sucrose, etc.

xi. *Colourants* Colouring agents are added to impart colour, elegance and to make the tablets easily identifiable. The colouring materials should be harmless, and only approved colours should be used. In solid preparations, the colouring agent is either mixed with dry powders or may be dissolved in a solution used for granulation. In liquid preparations, the colours are dissolved in the vehicle to give uniform colouration to the product; e.g., some natural colours are annatto, carotene, chlorophyll, curcumin, red and yellow oxides of iron. Some artificial colours are caramel, brilliant blue, naphthol blue, orange-G, and sunset yellow.

xii. *Coating agents* These are materials used to coat a formed tablet to protect against drug decomposition by atmospheric oxygen or humidity, to provide a desired release pattern for the drug substance after administration, to mask the taste and odour of the drug substance, or for aesthetic purposes. There are three types of coating: (a) sugar coating, (b) film coating, and (c) enteric coating.

a) Sugar coating is done using liquid glucose. This coating generally increases the weight of the tablet; it also masks the bitter taste of the drug and the additions.

b) Film coating is generally done by dissolving a solution of hydroxy propylmethyl cellulose, propylene glycol and a colourant, and then spraying it over the tablets in a rotating pan. The film is thin and plastic-like and there is no change in the weight, size or shape of the tablet.

c) Enteric coating is done using a solution of cellulose acetate phthalate or shellac. This coating is generally thick and prevents the dissolution and break-up of the tablet in the low acidic pH of the stomach, so that the tablet moves into the intestine unchanged. There, under the alkaline pH of the intestines, the enteric coating dissolves and the tablet breaks up. Usually, the enteric coatings are designed to dissolve at pH 4.8 or higher.

xiii. *Polishing agents* Tablets are polished with waxes to make them look attractive; e.g., carnuaba wax.

4.4 Classification

It is necessary to relate the drug substance and the disease state before the correct combination of drug and dosage form is made, as each disease or illness requires a specific type of drug therapy.

To have an overall understanding of formulations, it is essential to classify them into: i) route-wise dosage forms, and ii) form-wise dosage forms.

4.4.1 Route-wise dosage forms

Each route has its own demands and restrictions. The design of the drug delivery system through such routes has to cater to the specific needs of that route. Depending on the route of the administration of a drug, the formulations are broadly classified into: i) enterals, ii) parenterals, and iii) intradermal dosage forms (Fig. 4.1).

Route-wise dosage forms

Enterals (orals)	Parenterals	Intradermal
1. tablets	1. intramuscular	1. ointments
2. capsules	2. intravenous	2. creams
3. syrups	3. subcutaneous	
4. suspensions		

Fig. 4.1 *Classification of route-wise dosage forms.*

Enteral (oral) dosage forms are administered through the mouth. Oral dosage forms are meant for the placement of the drug into or through the gastrointestinal tract (GIT). It is a very significant route as it is a natural, uncomplicated, convenient and safe means for the transfer of hosts of material to the system, including food. The oral dosage form may be for local action on the oral mucosa or for systemic action.

Parenteral dosage forms They are meant for direct introduction of the drug into the blood, tissues, organs, etc. Though there are many parenteral routes, the intramuscular, intravenous, and subcutaneous are the primary routes.

Intradermal dosage forms are applied to the skin. They are meant for the absorption of the drug into the tissues and bloodstream. Transdermal patches for sustained but slow entry of drugs into the systemic circulation, across the cutaneous tissues, have been introduced recently.

4.4.2 Form-wise dosage forms

Depending on the nature of the dosage forms, formulations are classified as: a) solid, b) semi-solid, and c) liquid dosage forms. The further subclass of the form-wise dosage form is shown in Fig. 4.2.

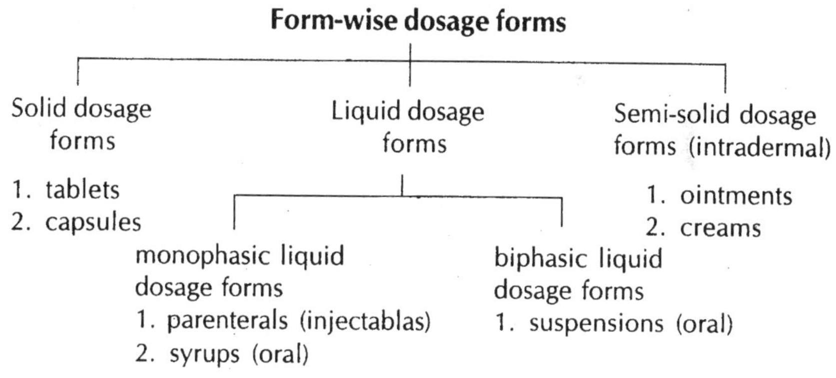

Fig. 4.2 *Classification of form-wise dosage forms.*

4.5 Solid dosage forms (enterals)

Tablets and capsules are the solid dosage forms containing the therapeutic agent/s with or without non-therapeutic agents. When therapeutic agents are to be administered orally in a dry form, tablets and capsules are most frequently used. They are effective and convenient for the patient to handle, identify, carry and administer. From a pharmaceutical standpoint, solid dosage forms are generally more stable than their liquid counterparts and thus are preferred for poorly stable drugs.

4.5.1 Tablets

Tablets are solid dosage forms of medicinal substances usually prepared with the aid of suitable pharmaceutical additives. These additives are diluents, binding agents, granulating agents, disintegrating agents, lubricants, colouring agents, flavouring agents, and sweetening agents (discussed in the earlier section).

For the preparation of good quality tablets, either the crystalline form or the granules of the ingredients are used rather than fine powders. The reasons for preferring granules over fine powders is as follows: (a) granules flow evenly through the hopper resulting in tablets of uniform weight, (b) granules are uniform so they cannot separate into layers, (c) in granules, colour distributes uniformly, and (d) finally granules are heavier, so they cannot flow out of the hopper.

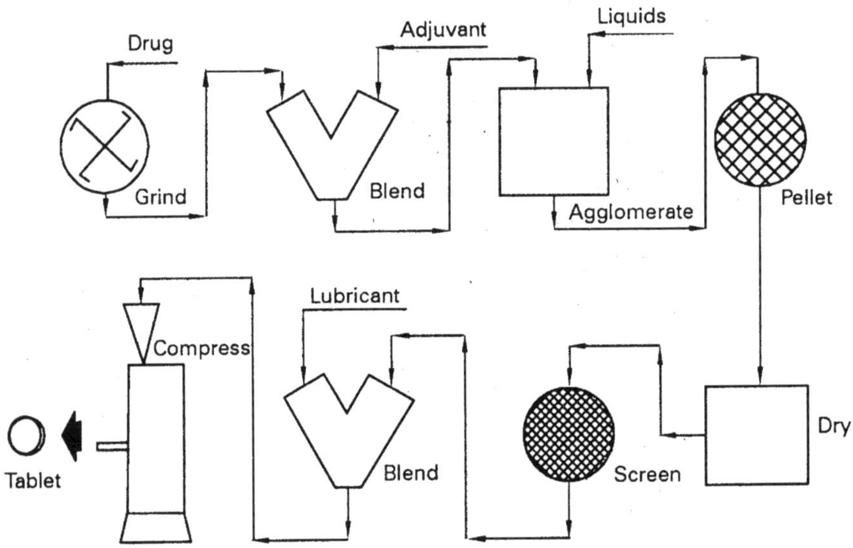

Fig. 4.3 *Flow diagram of the wet granulation method for the manufacture of tablets.*

The wet granulation method is widely used for the production of tablets. In this method, the powdered therapeutic agent is mixed along with additives like diluents, binding agents, and disintegrating agents. The mixture is then moistened with a sufficient amount of granulating agent (water or alcohol) to form a coherent mass. This coherent mass is passed through sieve No. 8 or 10 to get uniformly-sized granules. The wet granules so obtained are spread in thin layers and dried at 60°C in a hot air oven. The dried granules are passed through sieve No. 20 to get uniformly-sized granules. They are then mixed with the second portion of the disintegrating agent, lubricants and flavouring agents and finally the granules are compressed to form tablets in a metal die on a tablet press. The base of the die is a lower punch and above the die is an upper punch. When the upper punch is forced down upon the powder mix or granules (single punch press) or when the upper and lower punches are squeezed together (rotary press), the powder mix or granules are forced into a tablet. Tablet-making machines are single-punch machines, multi-punch machines, rotary tablet machines, double-rotary tablet machines, dry-coat tablet machines.

After the tablets are formed, they are coated. The purpose of tablet coating is to protect it from atmospheric effects, to make the tablet look more elegant, to improve its unpleasant taste and odour of the drug and to prevent its disintegration in stomach. The manufacturing procedure of ciprofloxacin hydrochloride is discussed below.

The composition of a tablet of the antibacterial drug, ciprofloxacin (containing 250 mg of ciprofloxacin), is shown in Table 4.1, i.e., 250 mg of ciprofloxacin in the form of hydrochloride salt weighing 290 mg.

Preparation of tablets The active ingredient (drug) and the additives required in the tablet formulation are weighed and mixed thoroughly. Generally, tablets are manufactured in batches of 1, 2, 3, 4 or 5 lakhs (e.g., to prepare 5 lakh tablets of ciprofloxacin 250 mg, 145 kg of ciprofloxacin hydrochloride (5,00,000 × 290 mg ciprofloxacin hydrochloride) is required. The common diluents used are lactose, microcrystalline cellulose, starch and powdered sucrose. The common disintegrating agents used are corn, potato starch, and polyvinyl pyrrolidone. The powdered

Table 4.1 *Composition of a 250 mg Ciprofloxacin Tablet*

Sl. No.	Component	Quantity	Nature of the additive
1.	Ciprofloxacin hydrochloride	290 mg	Drug
2.	Microcrystalline cellulose	20 mg	Binder, diluent, disintegrant, lubricant
3.	Lactose	20 mg	Diluent
4.	Cornstarch	20 mg	Binder and disintegrant
5.	Polyvinyl pyrrolidine	20 mg	Suspending and stabilizing
6.	Magnesium stearate	6 mg	Lubricant and glidant
7.	Sodium starch glycolate syrup	6 mg	Suspending and stabilizing agent
8.	Hydroxy propyl methylcellulose	6 mg	Binder
9	Titanium dioxide	3 mg	Colourant
	Total	400 mg	

mixture of all the ingredients is converted into free-flowing granules by the addition of the granulating agent (water or ethanol) and binding agents such as 10–20% aq. preparation of corn starch. The granules are sieved through no. 6 or 8 mesh sieves and to these granules a lubricant, such as talc or magnesium stearate, is added. The lubricant helps in the free flow of the granules and prevents the adhesion of the tablet to the die wall. The granules are now compressed into tablets using a steel die. The tablets are checked for weight variation, hardness and thickness before packing (Table 4.1).

Generic and trade names of drugs

Ciprofloxacin is the non-proprietory (generic) name. The generic name of a drug is proposed by the discoverer of the drug and is usually approved by the concerned drug authority of the country where it is discovered and registered. Generally, the Federal Drug Authority (FDA) approves the generic name of a drug in USA. Only the generic name is used in the chemical and medicinal literature of the drug and is different from its IUPAC or chemical abstracts (CA) nomenclature. A generic name should be: 1) short and distinctive in sound and spelling, so that it is memorable and not easily confused with the existing names of other drugs, and 2) indicate the general pharmacologic or therapeutic class into which the drug falls. Table 4.2 gives the generic names, therapeutic class, chemical class, and trade or brand names of some common drugs (see page 16).

Table 4.2 *Examples of some Generic and Trade Names of Drugs.*

	Generic name	Therapeutic class	Chemical structure	Trade/brand or proprietory name
E.g. 1.	Cipro**floxacin**	Antibacterial	Quinolone	Ciproplus-250 Ciprobid-250
	Nor**floxacin**	"	"	"
	Lomi**floxacin**	"	"	"
E.g. 2.	Peni**cillin** G	Antibacterial	β-lactam	Pfizerpen
	Amoxi**cillin**	"	"	Novamax, Mxgen
	Ampi**cillin**	"	"	Amcill, Polycillin
E.g., 3.	Capto**pril**	ACE inhibitor (antihypertension)	Peptide	Capotril
	Enala**pril**	"	"	Lexxel, Vaseretic, Enam
	Lisino**pril**	"	"	Prinivil, Prinzide

Drugs are generally sold under a trade name (or brand name or proprietory name), rather than by the generic name. Even the original discoverer of the drug sells it by a trade or brand name, which is short, catchy, easy to remember and contains a word indicating a portion of the generic name or the name of the manufacturer. Drugs that are not covered by the patent regulations are manufactured by companies other than the discoverer and formulated and sold with various trade or brand names. Ciprofloxacin is the generic name while Ciprabid-250 and Ciproplus-250 are the trade or brand names. The additives and diluents used by different formulators of a drug may vary slightly or largely, and is responsible for the slight differences in the biological effects produced by different brands of the same drug. This factor affects the acceptance by the patients as well as the sales of the drug. The sales of different brands of a drug also depend on the promotion through hospitals and doctors, the cost of the drug and attractiveness of packaging.

Table 4.3 *Examples of some of the Enteral Dosage Forms (Tablets)*

	Generic name	Trade name	Dosage	Therapeutic class
1.	Chlorpheniramine maleate	Aluma-drine	4, 8, 12 mg	Antihistamine
2.	Diazepam	Valium	2, 5, 10 mg	Sedative
3.	Haloperidol	Haldol	0.5, 1, 2, 5, 10 20 mg	Tranquillizer
4.	Ibuprofen	Motrin	300, 400, 600, 800mg	Analgesic
5.	Metronidazole	Flagyl	250, 500 mg	Anti-amoebic
6.	Propranolol HCl	Inderal	10, 20, 40, 60 mg	Antihypertension
7.	Tolbutamide	Orinase	250, 500 mg	Antidiabetic

4.5.2 Capsules

Mothes, a French pharmacy student in collaboration with a French pharmacist Dublanc, first invented the gelatin capsule in 1834.

Capsules are solid dosage forms, in which one or more therapeutic agent and/or additives are enclosed within a small shell or container, generally prepared from suitable forms of gelatin. Some of the advantages of capsules are: i) they are easy to administer because of their smooth and slippery nature, ii) enclosing a drug in a tasteless shell can mask its bitter and unpleasant taste, iii) they provide ease in dispensing a single dose.

There are two types of gelatin capsules in use. Depending on their formulation, the gelatin capsule shells are hard or soft. Hard gelatin capsules are used for filling solid substances, whereas soft gelatin capsules are used for filling semi-solids and liquid substances.

4.5.2.1 Hard gelatin capsules

They are made from a mixture of gelatin, water and sugar. They are clear, colourless and essentially tasteless. Gelatin is a product obtained from the partial hydrolysis of collagen obtained from the skin, white connective tissue, and bones of animals. As gelatin is soluble in hot water and in warm gastric fluids, a gelatin capsule readily dissolves and releases its contents. Also gelatin, being a protein, is digested and absorbed. Hard gelatin capsule shells are manufactured in two sections: the capsule body and the shorter cap. Capsule shells are available in various sizes and a suitable one is selected according to the amount of the medicament to be filled. Solid medicament is filled in the body of the capsule and the cap is placed over it. Capsule-making machines automatically remove the caps from empty capsules, fill the capsules with ingredients, replace the cap over the body and clean the capsules on the outside. Tamper-resistant capsule sealing is done, in which the contact areas of the capsules cap and body are wetted with a mixture of water and ethanol and then thermally bonded at 104° to 113°F. The filled and sealed capsules are cleaned and polished on the outside (Fig. 4.4).

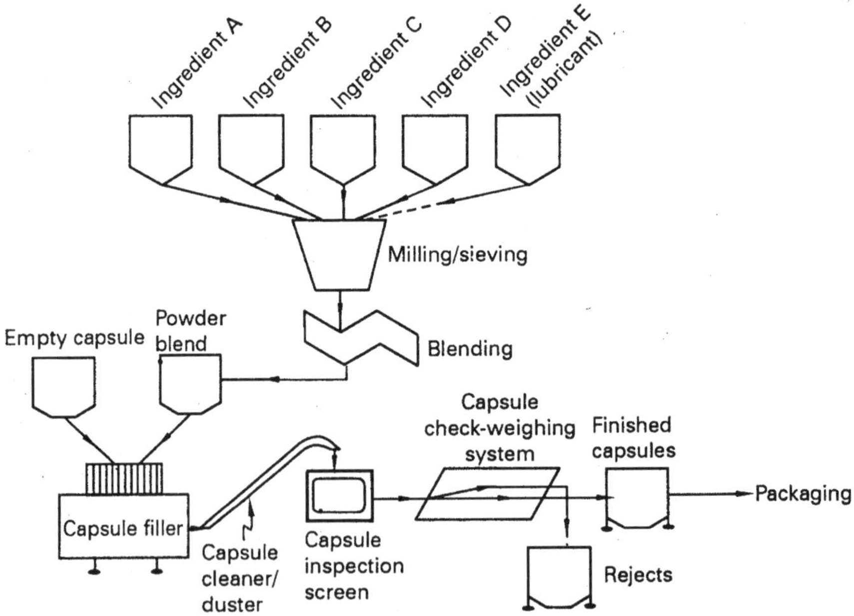

Fig. 4.4 *Flow diagram of the capsule manufacturing process.*

4.5.2.2 Soft gelatin capsules

Soft gelatin capsules are prepared from shells of gelatin to which glycerin or a polyhydric alcohol, such as sorbitol, has been added to render the gelatin elastic or plastic-like. Soft gelatin capsules are useful when it is necessary to seal the liquid therapeutic agent within the capsule. Soft gelatin capsules contain liquid drugs or drug solutions and volatile drug substances or drug materials which are especially susceptible to deterioration in the presence of air.

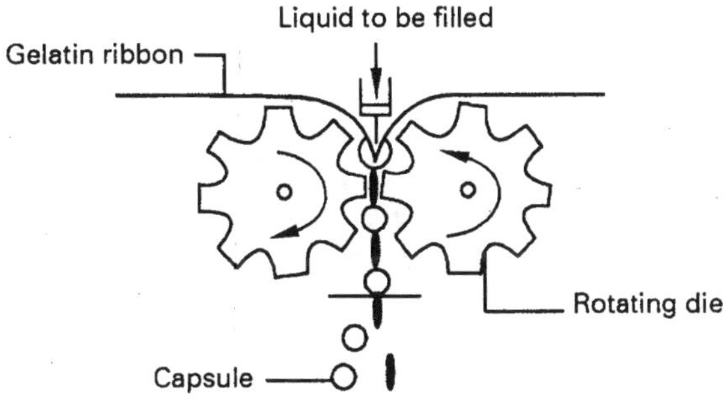

Fig. 4.5 *Flow diagram of the soft gelatin capsule manufacturing process.*

Most industrially-produced soft gelatin capsules are prepared by the rotary dry process (Fig. 4.5). The rotary machine is an automatic machine, in which two continuous sheets of gelatin are supplied to two die rolls rotating in opposite directions. As gelatin comes in between the rollers, the measured quantity of the therapeutic agent to be filled is injected through a metering device. The heat and the pressure exerted by the die rolls seals the two halves together. The capsules are then washed with naphtha solution and dried.

Finally, the capsules are subjected to certain tests that include: (i) weight variation test, (ii) contents uniformity test, and (iii) disintegration test. Examples of some commonly used capsule dosage forms are given in Table 4.4.

Table 4.4 *Examples of some Commonly Used Capsule Dosage Forms.*

Generic name	Brand Name	Dosage	Therapeutic Class
Amoxycillin	Wymox	250, 500 mg	Antibacterial
Ampicillin	Amcill	"	"
Cephalexin	Keflex	"	"
Diphenhydramine HCl	Benadryl	25, 50 mg	Antihistamine
Tetracyline HCl	Achyramycin	250, 500 mg	Antibacterial, Antibiotic

4.6 Liquid dosage forms

4.6.1 Parenterals (injectables)

The term 'parenteral' refers to the injectable routes of administration. This term has been derived from the Greek word "para" and "enteron", meaning "outside of the intestine", and denotes routes of administration other than the oral route. Parenterals should be sterile, *pyrogen-free, isotonic* and free from particles like dust and fibres. Parenteral preparations are used when rapid drug action is desired, as in emergency situations, when the patient is uncooperative, unconscious, or unable to accept or tolerate medication by the oral route, or when the drug itself is ineffective by other routes. The earliest injectable drug to receive official recognition was the hypodermic morphine solution.

Advantages Some of the advantages of the parentarals (injectables) are: i) for immediate physiological action of the drug in an emergency, the intravenous route of administration is followed, (ii) the modified form of the drug can be given by this route to slow down and prolong the action of the drug (Table 4.5), (iii) the drug can be administered parentarally when the patient is uncooperative, (iv) any amount of the drug can be administered, and (v) finally it is useful when the drugs are not well absorbed after oral administration.

Table 4.5 *Variation in the Time of Onset of Action for Different Dosage Forms*

Time of Onset of Action	Dosage Form
Seconds	Intravenous injection
Minutes	Intramuscular and subcutaneous injections, buccal tablets, aerosols, gases
Minutes to hours	Tablets, capsules, controlled-release tablets
Several hours	Enteric coated tablets
Days	Depot injections, implants

Disadvantages Some of the disadvantages of the parenterals (injectables) are: (i) a trained person is always required to administer the drugs except for insulin injections, which are commonly self-administered by diabetic patients, (ii) aseptic conditions and proper sterilization is necessary for parenteral products, (iii) administration through the wrong route, other than that intended, may prove fatal, and (iv) it is difficult to save a patient's life when an overdose is given.

Based on their physical characteristics, the parenterals (injectables) can be classified as: (i) solution form, (ii) emulsion form, (iii) suspension form, (iv) dry soluble products which are dissolved in a suitable solvent immediately before their administration, and (v) dry insoluble products, which are combined with a suitable vehicle before administration.

Parenterals can also be classified on the basis of the route of administration. However, injections are usually administered into a vein (intravenous or IV), into the skin (intramuscular or IM), intradermal, and subcutaneous (SC). The other routes are intra-articular (joints), intrasinovial (a joint fluid area), intra-arterial, intracardiac (into the heart), intrathecal (spinal fluid), and intraspinal.

Formulation of parenterals The formulation of parenterals requires a clear understanding of principles with regard to accuracy, measurements, cleanliness, and quality control of the product. It should have the minimum number of additives in the smallest possible quantities. These substances are vehicles and adjuvants.

Vehicles Generally, two types of vehicles are used, they are: i) aqueous, and ii) non-aqueous.

Aqueous vehicles Sterile water is used as a vehicle for a number of preparations, because it is well tolerated by the body and the safest to administer. The water must be free from pyrogens, volatile and non-volatile impurities.

Non-aqueous vehicles The commonly used non-aqueous vehicles are oils and alcohols. Oily vehicles are used when: (a) medicament is not stable in water, (b) delayed absorption is required, and (c) the drug is soluble in oil. Some examples are arachis oil, cottonseed oil, and sesame oil.

Adjuvants The minimum possible quantity of adjuvants are added to improve the quality and stability of the parenterals. They are: (i) solubulizing agents, (ii) stabilizers, (iii) buffers, e.g., citric acid and sodium citrate, (iv) antimicrobial agents, e.g., phenol (0.5% w/v) and cresol (0.3% w/v), (v) tonicity factors. All injections should be isotonic with blood plasma or with other body fluids, to reduce the pain and irritation of the injection in areas with many nerve endings. The isotonocity of a solution is adjusted by using dextrose, sodium chloride and sodium sulphate, and (vi) chelating agents, e.g., sodium or potassium salts of citric acid.

Preparation Once the formulation for a particular parenteral product is determined, including the selection of proper solvent or vehicles and additives, the pharmacist must follow rigid, aseptic procedures in preparing the injectable products. The manufacturing area must be free from bacteria and must have a filtered air supply, sterile manufacturing equipment and sterile clothing must be worn by the personnel in the area (good manufacturing practice or GMP).

In the preparation of parenteral solutions, the required ingredients are dissolved either in water for injection, or in one of the alternative solvents, or in a combination of solvents. The solutions are then filtered through a membrane- type filter and rapidly transferred to the final containers. The product is then sterilized, preferably by autoclaving, and samples of the finished products are tested for sterility and pyrogens. The sterile and pyrogen-free product is filled into ampoules/vials with the help of semi-automatic or automatic machines, under aseptic conditions. Finally, sealing is done by the fusion of glass in a hot flame or blast or torch, but nowadays automatic machines are available for large-scale production. The vials and bottles are sealed by rubber closure with the help of a vacuum, and then aluminum caps are further placed on them either by hand or by mechanical methods and labelled with instructions. Some of these products are listed in Table 4.6.

Table 4.6 *Examples of some of the Parenteral Dosage Forms (Injections)*

Injection	Physical form	Category	Administration
Cimetidine	Solution	Histamine H_2 antagonist	IM or IV
Dexamethasone sodium phosphate	Solution	Glucocorticoid, for cerebral edema and unresponsive shock	IM, IV also intra-articular
Heparin sodium	Solution	Anticoagulant	IV or SC
Hydromorphone-HCl	Solution	Narcotic analgesic used for moderate to severe pain	IV, SC or IM, or by slow IV
Procaine Penicillin G	Solution	Anti-infective	IM for moderate to severe infections due to penicillin G sensitive microorganisms
Verapamil - HCl	Solution	Calcium channel-blocking agent	Administered slowly through IV
Lidocaine - HCl	Solution	Cardiac depressant, anti-arrhythmic and also local anaesthetic	IV
Propranolol - HCl	Solution	β-adrenergic receptor blocking agent (management of hypertension)	IV

4.6.1.1 Total parenteral nutrition (TPN)

These solutions are generally administered by means of intravenous infusions to replenish body fluids and electrolytes, or to provide nutrition. They are usually administered in volumes of 100 ml to litre amounts and more, each day, by slow intravenous drip with or without controlled rate infusion system. TPN is given to increase the chance of a patient's survival in pre-operative and post-operative conditions. Generally, the TPN solution consists of a mixture of amino acids, lipid emulsions, electrolytes, and vitamins with trace elements. These solutions are packed in large single dose containers. Large-volume parenteral solutions are employed in *maintenance therapy* for patients entering into or recovering from surgery, or for the patient who is unconscious and unable to take fluids, electrolytes and nutrition orally. The solutions may also be utilized in *replacement therapy* for patients who have suffered a heavy loss of fluid and electrolytes.

Maintenance therapy When a patient is being maintained on parenteral fluids for a few days, simple solutions providing adequate amounts of sodium and potassium are generally sufficient. If a patient is on parenteral fluids for a large number of days, total parenteral nutrition must be implemented. Total nutrient admixtures (TNA) include carbohydrates, proteins, fats and electrolytes of trace elements. They are usually mixed in a single plastic intravenous bag for convenient administration.

Replacement therapy In the case of heavy loss of water and electrolytes, as in severe diarrhea or vomiting, greater than usual amounts of these materials may be initially administered and then maintenance therapy provided. Patients with AIDS, burns, or patients experiencing trauma are also candidates for replacement therapy.

Water requirement In normal individuals, the daily water requirement is the amount needed to replace normal and expected losses; for adults,it is about 25 to 40 ml/kg of the body weight. Generally, a patient with 50 kg of body weight may require 3.5 litres for replacement, plus 2.4 liters for maintenance. The patient who requires water generally requires nutrition and/or electrolytes. The parenteral administration of water is given as a solution with dextrose or electrolytes, where the solution has sufficient tonicity to protect the red blood cells from hemolyzing.

Electrolyte requirement Potassium and sodium are two important cations (electrolytes) present in the body. Potassium, the primary intracellular cation, is particularly important for normal cardiac and skeletal muscle functions. The daily intake of potassium is about 100 mEq and the daily loss is about 40 mEq. Thus, any replacement therapy should include a minimum of 40 mEq, and also the amount needed to replace additional losses. Potassium can be lost through excessive perspiration, repeated enemia, trauma, uncontrolled diabetes, diseases of the intestinal tract, surgical operations, etc. The symptoms of potassium loss include a weak pulse, faint heartbeats, falling blood pressure, and generalized weakness. An excess of potassium is also not good for health and may cause diarrhea, irritability, muscle cramps and pain.

In case of severe potassium deficiency, electrolyte replacement through the IV administration of potassium is usually employed. The usual additive dilution of potassium chloride is 40 mEq/litre of IV fluid, and the maximum infusion rate should not exceed 40 mEq/hour. Because of its potent ECG effects when infused, it is advisable to monitor the patient's ECG.

Sodium, the extracellular cation, is vital to maintain normal extracellular fluids. The average daily intake of sodium is 135 to 170 mEq, i.e., 8-10 mg of sodium chloride.

A low sodium level in the body may result from excessive sweating, the use of certain diuretics, or diarrhea. Fatigue, muscle weakness and convulsions are among the symptoms of excessive sodium loss. Symptoms of excess sodium are thirst, dry, sticky mucous membranes, flushed skin, elevated body temperature, lack of tears, etc. Chloride, the principle anion of the extracellular fluid, is usually paired with sodium. Chloride is also important for muscle contractions, balancing of fluid levels inside and outside the cells, and acid-base balance. The other electrolytes and minerals like calcium, magnesium and iron, which are lost from the body, are generally not required during short-term parenteral therapy.

Caloric requirement Patients requiring parenteral fluids are generally given 5% dextrose to reduce the caloric deficit that usually occurs in patients undergoing maintenance or replacement therapy. The use of dextrose also minimizes ketosis and the breakdown of proteins. The daily ingestion of at least 100 gm of glucose reduces this loss by itself.

4.6.2 Liquid oral dosage forms

The use of the liquid oral dosage form is justified on the basis of ease of administration and rapid absorption, for those individuals who cannot swallow solid dosage forms. Drugs are absorbed more rapidly in their dissolved state. Liquid oral dosage forms can be classified as: (i) monophasic liquid dosage form, and (ii) biphasic liquid dosage form.

i. *Monophasic liquid dosage forms* These are liquid formulations in which there is only one phase, e.g., solutions. They are: (a) liquids for internal administration, mixtures—*syrups* and elixirs, and (b) liquids meant for external administration or used on mucous membranes—gargles, mouthwashes, throat paints, douches, eardrops, liniments and lotions.

ii. *Biphasic liquid dosage forms* These are liquid formulations in which there are two phases, e.g., (a) *suspensions*, and (b) *emulsions*.

4.6.2.1 Syrups

Syrups are concentrated, aqueous preparations of medicinal substances with sugar or a sugar-substitute and with or without added flavouring agents.

Syrups are particularly effective in the administration of drugs for paediatric patients, as it provides a pleasant means of administering a liquid form of a disagreeable-tasting drug. Any water-soluble drug that is stable in aqueous solution may be added to a flavoured syrup.

Components of Syrups Most syrups contain: (i) the therapeutic agent in addition to purified water, (ii) sugar, usually sucrose, (iii) antimicrobial preservatives, (iv) flavourants, and v) colourants, and other stabilizers. Sucrose is the sugar most frequently employed in syrups. Most syrups contain a high proportion of sucrose, usually 60 to 80%, to resist microbial growth. In some cases, sugars are replaced with methoxycellulose and hydroxyethylcellulose, which are not hydrolyzed and absorbed into the bloodstream, and their use results in an excellent syrup-like vehicle for medication intended for diabetic patients.

Antimicrobial preservatives commonly used in syrups are benzoic acid and sodium benzoate (0.1 to 0.2%). Syrups are flavoured with synthetic flavourants or with naturally-occurring materials, such as volatile oils, e.g., orange oil, vanillin and others, to render a pleasant taste to the syrup. To make it more attractive, colouring agents like green with mint, brown with chocolate, etc. are added.

Table 4.7 *Components Used in the Preparation of Antihistamine Syrup.*

Components	Amounts
Chlorpheniamine maleate	0.4 g
Glycerine	25.0 ml
Syrup	83.0 ml
Sorbitol solution	60.0 ml
Sodium benzoate	1.0 g
Alcohol	60.0 ml
+ Colourants and Flavours, purified water to make upto	1 Litre

Preparation of Syrups In the preparation of syrups the therapeutic agent is mixed/heated/agitated with additives. For example, crocin syrup, albuterol sulphate syrup, and promethazine HCl syrup. The composition of an antihistamine syrup is (1 lit.) shown in Table 4.7 and other examples of syrups are given in Table 4.8.

Table 4.8 *Examples of some Commonly Used Syrups*

Components	Trade name	Therapeutic class
Chlorpromazine	Thorazine	Controls nausea and vomiting
Chlorpheniramine	Teldrin	"
Diphenhydramine	Benadryl	Controls cough

4.6.2.2 Suspensions

Suspensions may be defined as preparations containing finely-divided drug particles distributed uniformly throughout a vehicle, in which the drug exhibits a minimum degree of solubility. Suspensions are biphasic liquid dosage forms for oral administration like lotions for topical application to the skin, ophthalmic suspensions for the eyes, and sterile suspensions for injections.

The size of the dispersed phase is usually 0.5 to 5.0 mm, and is an important consideration in the formulation process. The suspension for topical application should have smaller-sized particles to cover a greater area of application and a faster rate of dissolution, to help in penetration. Injectable suspensions should have a particle size that can pass through the needle.

Suspensions are of two types: the suspensions which do not require reconstitution at the time of dispensing, are in (i) Ready-to-use form: here, the drug is already distributed through a liquid vehicle with or without a stabilizer and other additives. (ii) Dry powders: which need reconstitution at the time of usage. The product is generally a powder mixture containing the drug, suitable for suspending and dispensing agents (usually purified water), which on dilution and agitation results in the formation of a suspension suitable for administration. The drugs that are unstable in the vehicle if maintained for extended periods, are supplied as dry powder mixtures for reconstitution at the time of dispensing.

The reasons for preparing oral suspensions are several. Certain drugs are chemically unstable when in solution, but stable when suspended. In such instances, suspensions ensure chemical stability. For many patients, the liquid form is preferred to the solid form of the same drug because of the ease of swallowing liquids and the flexibility in the administration of a range of doses. The disadvantage of the disagreeable taste of certain drugs when given in solution form is overcome when the drug is administered as undissolved particles of a suspension. This is particularly advantageous for infants, children and the aged.

The characteristics of a good suspension are: (i) it should be chemically stable, (ii) the sediment produced on standing should be easily redispersed, (iii) the viscosity should be such that the preparation can be easily poured, (iv) suspensions meant for internal use must be palatable, and suspensions for external use must be free from gritty particles.

Ready-to-use suspensions They are of two types: (a) suspensions containing diffusible solids, and (b) suspensions containing indiffusible solids.

a) *Suspensions containing diffusible solids* Solids which are insoluble in water but readily mix with water, and remain suspended throughout the liquid for sufficiently long time after shaking, are known as diffusible solids; e.g., calcium carbonate, magnesium trisilicate. To prepare these formulations the medicament is finely powdered, and is mixed with enough vehicle to form a smooth cream; an additional vehicle is added to make it pourable. It is passed through a piece of muslin to strain any foreign particles. After making it up to the required volume with the vehicle, it is bottled with a cork and labelled with a direction "Shake the bottle before use".

b) *Suspension containing indiffusible solids* A solid is regarded as indiffusible when it does not remain uniformly distributed in the vehicle for a sufficiently long time; e.g., aspirin, phenobarbitone, hydrocortisone, calamine. To suspend the drug, certain thickening and wetting agents are added. Thickening agents are hydrophilic colloids that form colloidal dispersions with water and increase the viscosity of continuous phase, so that the particles remain suspended for a sufficiently long time and it becomes easy to measure an accurate dosage; e.g., gum acacia, tragacanth, starch, cellulose derivatives, aluminum hydroxide. Wetting agents are added to prepare suspensions of desired quality by reducing the interfacial tension between the solid particles and liquid medium; e.g., alcohol in tragacanth mucilage, glycerin and glycols in sodium alginate dispersion. In preparing these suspensions, the pharmacist must be acquainted with the characteristics of both the dispersed phase and dispersion medium. The dispersed phase is readily "wetted" by the addition of the vehicle; in this case, the vehicle also acts as a wetting agent. The drugs that are not penetrated easily by the vehicle are to be wetted first using wetting agents like alcohols, glycerins and other hygroscopic liquids. Once the powder is wetted, the dispersion medium (containing colourants, flavourants, and preservatives) is added in portions to the powder, and the mixture is thoroughly blended before the subsequent addition of the vehicle. Finally, suitable preservatives are added, and they are packed in wide mouthed containers, which have adequate air space above the liquid to permit shaking and ease of pouring. It is labelled with a direction "Shake the bottle before use".

ii *Dry powders* These need reconstitution at the time of usage. There are a number of formulations in the form of dry powder mixtures or granules, which are intended to be suspended in water or in some other vehicle prior to usage; e.g., magnesia and alumina oral suspension, erythromycin estolate oral suspension, methyldopa oral suspension, amoxicillin for oral suspension – USP, ampicillin for oral suspension – USP, cephalexin for oral suspension – USP.

4.7 Semi-solid dosage forms (intradermal)

Many pharmaceutical agents meant for topical application to intact skin or broken skin or to mucous membranes, have been presented in the form of semi-solids of viscous consistency. They have been designated as ointments, creams, pastes, etc. and used mainly as a protective screen or emollient for the skin.

4.7.1 Ointments

Ointments are meant for external application to the skin and mucous membranes, and the therapeutic agent present in it is absorbed systemically. Modern day ointments serve this purpose and also carry therapeutic agents for percutaneous absorption (through the skin) and action on the deeper layers of tissues as well. Accordingly, they are classified as: (i) epidermic—meant for action on the skin, (ii) endodermic—meant for action on deeper layers of cutaneous tissues, and (iii) diadermic—meant to penetrate deep and release the therapeutic agent to the body fluids.

All ointments consist of a base which chiefly acts as a carrier for the therapeutic agent. The nature of the base also controls its performance. Therefore, the selection of the ointment base is a very important aspect of formulation. The affinity between the drug and the base determines the release rate of the drug. Substances with lower solubility are released more easily. The ointment bases are classified into four general groups: (a) Oleaginous bases, e.g, hydrocarbons, vegetable oils, hydrogenated and sulphated oils, (b) Absorption bases, e.g, cottonseed oil, white vaseline, and c) Water-soluble bases, e.g, polyethylene glycols.

Preparation Ointments are prepared using two general methods: (i) incorporation, and (ii) fusion. The method for a particular preparation depends upon the nature of the ingredients.

i) *Incorporation method* In this method, the ingredients are mixed thoroughly by various methods until a uniform preparation has been attained. On a small scale, the pharmacist mixes the components using a mortar and pestle. If the therapeutic agent is solid, it is dissolved in a suitable solvent and the base is added and uniformly mixed. In large-scale preparations, the ointment is coarsely prepared in powerful ointment and paste-mixers. Mechanical ointment-roller mills force coarsely-formed ointments through moving stainless steel rollers, resulting in the formation of products that are smooth and uniform in composition and texture.

ii) *Fusion method* Here, all or some of the ingredients of the ointment are combined by being melted together and cooled with constant stirring until they congeal and become solid. The components that are not melted are generally added to the congealing mixture as it is being cooled and stirred. Heat-labile substances and volatile substances are added when the temperature of the mixture is low. Many medicated ointments, which do not lend themselves well to mixtures by the incorporation method, are prepared by the fusion method. Most of the ointments must be stored below 30° C to prevent softening and even liquifying of the base; e.g., gentamycin ointment, neomycin sulphate ointment, nystatin ointment, and monobenzene ointment.

4.7.2 Creams

Creams are classified under dermatological dosage forms, intended for application to the skin. Creams are defined as "Viscous liquid or semi-solid emulsions of either the oil-in-water or the water-in-oil type". They are usually employed as emollients which smooth the skin or as medicated applications to the skin. Creams are applied to the skin either for their physical effects, that is, for their ability to act as skin protectants, lubricants, emollients, drying agents, etc., or for the specific effect of the medicinal agent(s) present. Creams are preferred to ointments due to their easier spreadability and the fact that they are easier to remove than ointments.

The absorption of substances from outside the skin to positions beneath the skin, including entrance into the bloodstream, is referred to as percutaneous absorption. The pharmaceutical absorption of a medicinal substance present in the transdermal therapeutic system or in a dermatological preparation, depends not only upon the physical and chemical properties of the medicinal substance, but also upon its behavior when placed in the vehicle, and the conditions of the skin. Although a pharmaceutical vehicle may not penetrate the skin nor actually carry the medicinal substance through the skin, the vehicle does influence the rate and degree of penetration of a medicinal agent; e.g., nystatin cream, miconozole nitrate, benzocain cream and gentamycin sulphate.

The other non-medicated creams are vanishing creams, cold creams, cleansing creams, foundation creams, and moisturising creams.

Vanishing Creams These are generally oil-in-water emulsions, containing large percentage of water and stearic acid. When these creams are applied to the skin, the water evaporates leaving behind a thin residual film of the stearic acid. A vanishing cream contains oil, stearic acid, alkali and water. A good vanishing cream is always a pearly-white, shining product, which, on application, gives a thin white film of free stearic acid.

Cold Creams Cold creams are semi-solid, white, water-in-oil emulsion prepared with cetyl esters wax, white wax, mineral oil, sodium borate and purified water. When it is applied to the skin, a cooling effect is produced due to the slow evaporation of the water present in it. Further, the presence of water in the base is useful because the occlusive (blocking) external phase traps the water onto the skin and enhances skin moisturization.

Cleansing Creams Cleansing creams are used to remove facial make-up. These creams form an emollient on the skin, which is protective in dry skin conditions. These are basically cold creams with a detergent for cleansing action. Cleansing creams require oils to dissolve unwanted material on the skin.

Foundation Creams They are used to provide a smooth emollient base for the application of cosmetics and powder. They also act as a skin protective to prevent the damage caused by environmental factors like the sun or wind. These creams contain fatty materials, stearic acid, sodium hydroxide, glycerin, emulsifying agents and surfactants.

Moisturising Creams Dry skin conditions can be corrected by these creams and they are usually applied at night. The uses of moisturising creams are that they protect against bacteria, give a fresh and natural appearance to the skin, help to preserve the skin, soften and maintain the skin's moisture content. They contain materials like glycerin, sorbitol, propylene glycol, mineral oil, lipophilic substances, vegetable oil, and lanolin.

QUESTIONS

I. Main Questions

1. Define pharmaceutics? Why do we convert drugs into formulations?
2. What are additives/excipients/adjuvants? What is their role in formulations.
3. Write the classification of formulations and briefly explain.
4. What are solid dosage forms? Write a short note on tablets, with examples.
5. What is the generic name and trade name? Explain with examples. Write a short note on capsules, with examples.
6. Write a brief note on parenterals (injections). Explain the advantages and disadvantages of parenterals?
7. What is total parentaral nutrition?
8. Classify liquid oral dosage forms. Explain syrups with examples.
9. Write a short note on suspensions with examples.
10. What are intradermal dosage forms? Write a note on ointments with examples.
11. What are different types of creams? Explain with examples.

II. Fill in the blanks with suitable answers.

1. In the manufacture of a tablet, titanium dioxide is used as a _____.
2. Captopril is __________ name of an antihypertensive drug.
3. Parenterals administered as _______ .
4. An ointment is an ________ dosage form.

III. Match the following.

Column 1	Column 2
1. Penicillin G	(a) binder, disintegrant
2. Vanishing cream	(b) lubricant
3. Starch	(c) polishing agent
4. Colcuim stearate	(d) intradermal dosage
5. Carnuba wax	(e) parenteral

Answers to objective questions

II. 1. Colourant 2. Generic 3. Injections 4. Intradermal

III. 1-e; 2-d; 3-a; 4-b; 5-c

Bibliography

1. Agarwal, O.P., *Synthetic Organic Chemistry*, Gel Publishing House, Meerut.
2. Ananthanarayan, R. and Paniker, Jayaram C.K., *Textbook of Microbiology* (5th Edition), Orient Longman, Chennai.
3. Ansel, Howard C., Popovich, Nichalas G. and Allen, Lloyd V. Jr., *Pharmaceutical Dosage Forms and Drug Delivery Systems* (6th Edition), B.I. Waverly Pvt. Ltd., New Delhi.
4. Berkow, R., Beers, Mark H., and Fletcher, Andrew J. (Ed.), *The Merck Manual of Medical Information,* Home Edition, Pocket Books, USA.
5. Biswas, S.B. and Biswas, Amita, *An Introduction to Viruses* (3rd Edition) Vikas Publishing House Pvt. Ltd., New Delhi.
6. Burgen, A.S.V. and Mitchell, J.F., *Gaddum's Pharmacology* (9th Edition), Oxford University Press, 1985.
7. Chatwal, Gurdeep R., *Synthetic Drugs*, Himalaya Publishing House, Bombay.
8. Foye, William O., Lemke,Thomas L., and Williams, David A., *Principles of Medicinal Chemistry* (4th Edition) B.I. Waverly Pvt. Ltd., New Delhi.
9. Goodman and Gilman, *Clinical Pharmacology.*
10. Grahame-Smith, D.G. and Aronson J.K., *Oxford Textbook of Clinical Pharmacology and Drug Therapy* (2nd Edition) Oxford University Press, Oxford.
11. Kar, Ashutosh, *Medicinal Chemistry*, Wiley Eastern Limited, New Delhi, 1993.
12. Laurence D.R. and Bennett P.N., *Clinical Pharmacology.*
13. Mittal B.M., *A Textbook of Pharmaceutical Formulation,* (6th Edition) Vallabh Prakashan, New Delhi, 1997.
14. Nand, Pratibha and Khar, Roop K., *Pharmaceutical Dispensing*, New Delhi, 1995.
15. Parimoo, P., *A Textbook of Medicinal Chemistry*, CBS Publishers and Distributors, New Delhi.
16. Powar, C.B., *Cell Biology*, Himalaya Publishing House, Bombay.
17. Sarma, P.D., *Microbiology and Plant Pathology,* Rastogi Publications, Meerut.
18. Satoskar, R.S., Bhadarkar, S.D. and Ainpure, S.S., *Pharmacology and Pharmacotherapeutics,* Vols. **1** & **2** (14th Edition) Popular Prakasham, Bombay.
19. Tierney, Lawrence M. Jr., Mc Phee, Stephen J., and Papadakis, Maxine A. (Ed.) *Current Medical Diagnosis and Treatment* (35th Edition), USA, 1996.

Glossary

ACE inhibitor Angiotensin Converting Enzyme inhibitor.

Afferent Nerves carrying sensation towards the brain.

Allergen A substance that causes an allergic reaction.

Allergy A disorder in which the body becomes hypersensitive to a particular antigen (the antigen is called allergen).

Analgesic A pain-reliever.

Androgen A male sex hormone.

Anemia A reduction in the quantity of haemoglobin (oxygen-carrying pigment). It may be due to the loss of blood (hemorrhagic anemia), or deficiency of iron (iron-deficiency anemia), or increased destruction of RBC (hemolytic anemia).

Ankylosing spondylitis inflammation of the spine and large joints, resulting in stiffness and pain.

Antibacterial A substance that prevents the growth of, or kills, bacteria.

Antibiotic A substance produced by microorganisms (mould or bacteria) that inhibits the growth of,or even destroys, other microorganisms.

Antibody A special type of blood protein that is synthesized by lymphocytes in response to the presence of a particular antigen.

Anti-emetic A drug that prevents vomiting (such drugs are also used to counter nausea).

Antigen A substance that the body identifies as foreign or potentially dangerous.

Anti-inflammatory A drug that inhibits inflammation.

Antipyretic A fever-reducing drug.

Asthma A disease characterized by difficulty in breathing (resulting from a paroxysmal attack of bronchospasms).

Bactericidal A substance that kills bacteria.

Bacteriostatic A substance that supresses the further growth of bacteria.

Beriberi The disease caused by a deficiency of thiamine (Vitamin B_1).

Broad-spectrum antibiotic An antibiotic that acts against a wide variety of microorganisms.

Cell membrane The outermost part of the cell made up of lipids and proteins.

Cell The basic structural unit of a living organism.

Cephalosporins Antibiotic agents which are structurally related to penicillin.

Chemotherapy Control or cure of infectious diseases caused by pathogens, by the use of chemicals

Cirrhosis of the liver (hepatocirrhosis) Condition where some cells of the liver die and are replaced by hard fibrous tissue.

Coenzyme A substance that binds to the protein part of an enzyme (apoenzyme), to make the functioning of an enzyme complete.

Cooley's anaemia (Thalassaemia) Hereditary type of anaemia due to a defect in the production of haemoglobin.

Dermatitis Inflammation of the skin, due to different reasons. This may result from direct irritation or allergic reaction by a substance that is in contact with the skin. The skin becomes red or itchy or small blisters may develop.

Dispersed phase, dispersion medium, suspension In the preparation of suspensions, the substance distributed is referred to as the dispersed phase and the vehicle is known as dispersion medium. The dispersed system is called suspension. The dispersed phase is usually made up of solid materials, which are insoluble in the dispersion medium.

Effector Special nerve ending in muscles or glands which is activated to produce contraction or secretion.

Enzyme A biological catalyst; it is a protein.

Estrogen A female sex hormone.

Expectorant A drug that increases respiratory tract secretions, lowers their viscosity and promotes removal.

Fats Esters derived from glycerol and fatty acids (triglycerides).

Fermentation A yeast-mediated process in which alcohol is produced.

Hemorrhage (bleeding) Escape of blood from a ruptured blood vessel, internally or externally.

Hormone A chemical messenger secreted by the endocrine glands in the body.

Hydrophilic Water-soluble.

Isotonic A solution is known as isotonic when its osmotic pressure is equal to the osmotic pressure of the blood plasma.

Liphophillic Fat-soluble.

Lumbago Low backache (severe lumbago is a sudden onset of backache while bending or lifting).

Malignant melanoma Dark tumour which develops on the skin, caused by exposure to strong sunlight.

Metabolism The sum of biochemical transformations that occur in living systems. It includes: (i) anabolism—synthesis of large molecules from smaller ones, and (ii) catabolism—degradation of larger molecules into smaller ones.

Motor nerves Nerves which carry impulses from the brain to the muscles and cause voluntary movement.

Mucoproteins Polymers in which amino sugars are combined with proteins.

Muscular dystrophy Any one of a group of muscle diseases, in which the affected muscle fibres degenerate and are replaced by fatty tissues.

Nausea A feeling that one is about to vomit.

Nephrotic syndrome Disease that affect the kidneys resulting in prolonged loss of protein through urine, decreased protein levels of the blood (especially albumin), and retention of excess salt and water in the body.

Nutrients The essential chemical ingredients of food, necessary for maintaining good health and energy, to promote growth, etc. (carbohydrates, proteins, fats, vitamins, minerals and water are the six classes of nutrients).

Oedema An excess accumulation of fluid in the body tissues beneath the skin (commonly known as dropsy).

Pathogen A disease-causing microbe.

Pellagra A disease that may be caused due to the deficiency of niacin (vitamin B_3); the symptoms are diarrhea, dermatitis, and dementia (loss of memory, mental confusion).

Pernicious anemia A disease due to the deficiency of vitamin B_{12}; characterized by the failure to produce RBC.

Posology Study of doses of medicine.

Prostaglandins Hormone-like compounds in the body that are involved in the increase of blood pressure, the contraction of smooth muscles, and other physiological processes such as pain management.

Pyrogens Pyrogens are fever-producing organic substances arising from microbial contamination, and are responsible for many of the febrile (fever) reactions that occur in patients following intravenous injections.

Rheumatism A disorder in which aches and pains occur in the muscles and joints.

Rheumatoid arthritis Pain and stiffness in the joints and muscles with inflammation, especially in the hands and feet.

Rickets A disease in children caused due to the deficiency of vitamin D, associated with malformed bones (softer than normal).

Salicin A glycoside derived from glucose and salicylic acid.

Sciatia A pain felt down the back and the outside of the thigh, foot and leg.

Scurvy A disease caused due to the deficiency of vitamin C (symptoms may involve swollen legs, spots of blood over the skin, stinking mouth with rotten gums).

Sickle-cell anaemia Hereditary condition where an abnormal red-blood cell shaped like a sickle, due to an abnormal haemoglobin, blocks the circulation causing anaemia.

Skeletal muscles Muscles which are attached to bones and are responsible for posture and movement.

Smooth muscles Involuntary muscles.

Testosterone Male sex hormone.

Vitamins A class of nutrients / dietary factors that are not biosynthesized by the human body (except D_2), and are supplied through diet.

Xerophthalmia A disease that is caused due to the deficiency of retinol; characterized by dry and lustreless eyeballs (this may eventually progress to blindness).

Index